Guided Meditation and Yoga

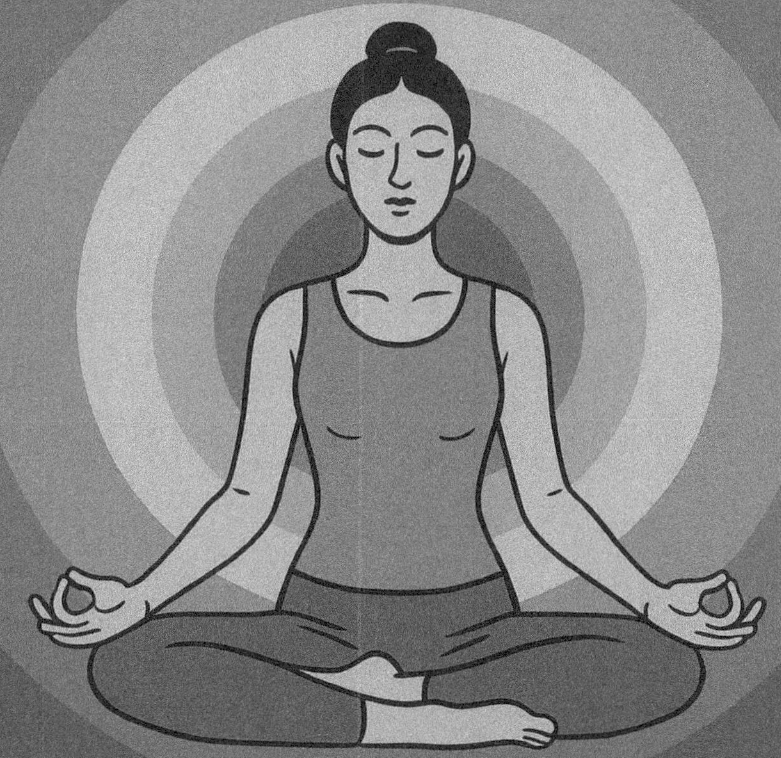

Jagdish Krishanlal Arora

Guided Meditation and Yoga

By

Jagdish Krishanlal Arora
techbagg@outlook.com

Also by Jagdish Krishanlal Arora

Table of Contents

Cultivate Patience and Persistence

Transcendental Meditation (TM)

Zen Meditation (Zazen)

Vipassana Meditation

Chakra Meditation

Guided Visualization

Body Scan Meditation

Sound Bath Meditation

Body-Oriented Meditation (e.g., Yoga, Tai Chi, Qigong):

Compassion Meditation (Tonglen)

Body-Observation Meditation (Vipassana)

Nada Yoga (Sound Yoga)

Exercise and Physical Activity

Social Support and Connection

Cognitive Behavioral Therapy (CBT)

Self-Compassion and Acceptance

Nature and Ecotherapy

Creative Expression

Integrate Meditation into Daily Life

Reduce stress, anxiety, and depression

Improve focus and concentration

Introduction to Meditation and Yoga

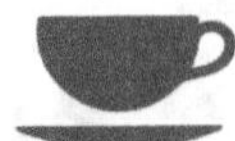

THE MULTITUDE OF HOLISTIC practices, including meditation, yoga, physical therapy exercises, gym workouts, swimming, and various other methods, harmoniously converge to unlock a treasure trove of physical, mental, and emotional benefits, culminating in a profound sense of well-being and vitality. In the fast-paced and often hectic world we inhabit, these practices serve as sanctuaries of solace, empowering individuals to shed the burdens of tension, stress, and anxiety, and to embrace a more positive, resilient, and energetic existence. With unwavering commitment and dedication, practitioners can pave the way towards reducing illness and diseases, forging a path towards a vibrant and holistic lifestyle.

Meditation, a timeless art of stilling the mind and cultivating mindfulness, has emerged as a transformative practice to navigate the complexities of modern living. Through the gentle guidance of meditation, individuals can detach from the incessant stream of thoughts, finding refuge in the stillness of the present moment. As the mind settles, tension and stress begin to dissipate, replaced by a sense of inner calm and tranquillity. By fostering awareness of their thoughts and emotions, practitioners develop the ability to respond to life's challenges with equanimity and grace, fostering a more positive and constructive outlook. Similarly, yoga, an ancient science of harmonizing the body, mind, and spirit, offers a tapestry of physical postures, breathwork, and meditation techniques. These practices cultivate flexibility, strength, and balance, while simultaneously nurturing a profound connection with the inner self. The fluidity of yoga postures, coupled with conscious breathing, enhances energy flow and revitalizes the body. Moreover, the meditative aspects of yoga anchor practitioners to the present moment, mitigating stress and fostering emotional resilience. The amalgamation of physical and mental practices in yoga enables individuals to develop an innate awareness of their bodies, thus preventing injuries and promoting overall well-being.

Physical therapy exercises (PT) serve as vital rehabilitative tools, aiding individuals in regaining strength, flexibility, and functionality after injuries or surgeries. The tailored exercises, designed to target specific areas of concern, not only restore physical prowess but also contribute to emotional healing. As individuals reclaim control over their bodies, the burden of stress and anxiety diminishes, replaced by a sense of empowerment and progress. The guidance and support of physical therapists play an integral role in optimizing the benefits of these exercises, ensuring safe and effective recovery.

Venturing into the realm of gyms, these vibrant spaces offer an array of fitness activities, catering to diverse preferences and goals. Engaging in regular gym workouts ignites the release of endorphins, the body's natural mood-enhancing chemicals, leading to a surge in positivity and a reduction in stress. Strength training, cardiovascular exercises, and aerobic routines build endurance and improve cardiovascular health, fostering a sense of vitality and overall fitness. Moreover, the social aspect of gym environments fosters camaraderie and support, nurturing a positive and motivating atmosphere for individuals striving towards their wellness goals.

Incorporating swimming into one's routine unlocks the wondrous benefits of low-impact aerobic exercise. As individuals glide through the water, they engage multiple muscle groups, promoting strength, flexibility, and coordination. Swimming is renowned for its capacity to instil a sense of relaxation and tranquillity, diminishing stress and anxiety. The rhythmic nature of swimming strokes and the immersive experience in water facilitate a meditative state, encouraging individuals to connect with the serenity within. Additionally, swimming is accessible to people of all ages and fitness levels, making it an inclusive and enjoyable activity.

Beyond these practices, various other methods contribute to the holistic tapestry of well-being. Engaging in outdoor activities, such as hiking, biking, or nature walks, fosters a sense of grounding and appreciation for the natural world, further reducing stress and promoting positivity. Creative pursuits, such as art, music, or writing, serve as therapeutic outlets, allowing individuals to express their emotions and foster a sense of fulfilment. The healing properties of spending time with animals, known as pet therapy, provide solace and comfort, reducing feelings of anxiety and loneliness.

The amalgamation of these practices in daily life extends far beyond mere physical fitness. As individuals integrate meditation, yoga, PT exercises, gym workouts, swimming, and other methods into their routines, they forge a path towards inner harmony and emotional equilibrium. The cultivation of mindfulness through meditation and yoga empowers individuals to navigate challenges with poise, embracing a positive and solution-oriented mindset. The resilience built through physical practices strengthens the body's ability to cope with stress, reducing the impact of external pressures on mental health. Moreover, the interplay of these practices nurtures a holistic approach to health, fostering a symbiotic relationship between the mind and the body. The physical benefits of improved cardiovascular health, increased flexibility, and enhanced muscular strength are mirrored by the mental benefits of reduced anxiety, improved focus, and heightened emotional well-being. The dynamic interconnection between the mind and body amplifies the overall sense of vitality and energy.

Furthermore, the implementation of these practices offers a host of preventive benefits, supporting the immune system and guarding against various diseases. The reduction of stress and anxiety fortifies the immune response, contributing to better overall health. Regular exercise, combined with the healing properties of meditation and yoga, lowers the risk of chronic conditions such as heart disease, diabetes, and obesity. Additionally, the positive impact of these practices on sleep quality enhances the body's ability to regenerate and heal, promoting overall wellness.

As individuals immerse themselves in these practices, the boundaries between the physical, mental, and emotional realms begin to blur, revealing the interconnectedness of the human experience. The pursuit of holistic well-being transcends the limitations of fragmented approaches, encouraging individuals to embrace an integrated approach to health. The interweaving of meditation, yoga, PT exercises, gym workouts, swimming, and other methods creates a symphony of well-being, wherein each practice harmonizes with the others, reinforcing their transformative potential.

In the profound journey towards holistic well-being, the human experience becomes a canvas for self-discovery and growth. As individuals delve deeper into the sacred sanctuary of meditation and yoga, they uncover the power of self-awareness and self-compassion. The gentle guidance of physical therapy exercises nurtures patience and resilience, instilling the wisdom of gradual progress and healing. The camaraderie and support found in gym environments nurture a sense of belonging and community, fostering a positive and uplifting atmosphere. As individuals immerse themselves in the immersive serenity of swimming and the healing embrace of various other methods, they embark on a journey of self-care and inner exploration. The tapestry of these practices unravels the transformative power of self-love, inviting individuals to prioritize their well-being and embrace a more balanced and holistic lifestyle.

In the embrace of meditation, yoga, PT exercises, gym workouts, swimming, and other methods, individuals can navigate the challenges of modern life with grace, resilience, and equanimity. As they shed the layers of tension, stress, and anxiety, they emerge as more vibrant, empowered, and self-aware beings. In the canvas of holistic well-being, individuals unveil the masterpiece of their own lives, embodying the essence of vitality, serenity, and harmony. As they intertwine these practices into the fabric of their daily existence, they embark on a lifelong journey towards wholeness, authenticity, and profound well-being. In this tapestry of self-discovery, they become the weavers of their own destinies, crafting a symphony of inner peace, joy, and transformation.

Relation of Meditation and Yoga

MEDITATION AND YOGA have been praised for their numerous benefits on both the mind and body. They have shown remarkable efficacy in mitigating stress, managing various illnesses, and fostering holistic well-being. Meditation is just another form of self-hypnosis. While self-hypnosis is difficult and requires external help, meditation can be done easily and is not as deep as hypnosis. No matter how deep you go into meditation, you will not achieve the same effects of calm and peace as you get in self-hypnosis and you only get an upper effect. Achieving a deep hypnotic state in meditation is impossible and it is not achieved even after several years of doing meditation as it requires a calm and noiseless atmosphere. To understand the difference in between meditation and self- hypnosis you need to go into self-hypnosis once which stills the mind and is like an instant relief.

The purpose of both is the same only meditation is done consciously when you are mostly awake and attaining deep meditation is itself self-hypnosis. The final stage of meditation is self-hypnosis through thoughts rather than receiving instructions from someone else or giving suggestions to yourself. In meditation you give suggestions to yourself using thoughts in your own mind. In self-hypnosis you get the effect in minutes which will take you years of meditation to get the same effect.

Yoga and physical exercise are the same. The only difference is that yoga has several postures which can twist our body and muscles and stretch them to the extreme possible. This helps to release the tension in the muscles and joints and shift the pain sections in the blood to other parts of the body and improve the blood circulation. Yoga also helps to remove stiffness and stuck body parts and joints. The same effect can be obtained by normal exercises taught in schools, but we find them difficult to do and for us Yoga is something unique we want to explore.

Below are some of the key benefits of meditation and yoga:

Stress Reduction: Both meditation and yoga are potent tools in reducing stress levels. Meditation promotes relaxation by calming the mind and reducing the production of stress hormones like cortisol. Similarly, yoga's focus on breath control and mindfulness encourages a sense of tranquillity, easing tension and promoting emotional balance.

Improved Mental Health: Regular practice of meditation and yoga can have a positive impact on mental health. They have been shown to reduce symptoms of anxiety and depression, enhance emotional regulation, and increase feelings of happiness and contentment.

Enhanced Focus and Concentration: Meditation cultivates mindfulness, which enhances cognitive functions such as focus, attention, and memory. Yoga, through its meditative aspects, helps individuals attain better concentration and mental clarity.

Better Sleep Quality: Meditation has been linked to improved sleep patterns, making it an effective remedy for insomnia and sleep disturbances. Certain yoga practices, such as restorative yoga, can also aid in relaxation and promote better sleep.

Physical Flexibility and Strength: Yoga's diverse asanas (postures) target different muscle groups, promoting flexibility and strength. The practice helps improve joint health, balance, and overall physical fitness.

Cardiovascular Health: Both meditation and yoga have been associated with cardiovascular benefits. Meditation reduces blood pressure and heart rate, while yoga can help improve blood circulation and overall heart health.

Pain Management: Meditation and certain yoga techniques have been used as complementary therapies for managing chronic pain conditions, such as arthritis and lower back pain. They can increase pain tolerance and alter the perception of pain.

Immune System Boost: Regular meditation and yoga practice have been linked to improved immune function. Reduced stress levels and enhanced relaxation contribute to a stronger immune system, making the body more resilient to illnesses.

Hormonal Balance: Meditation and yoga can influence hormonal balance, leading to reduced stress hormone levels and increased production of feel-good hormones like serotonin and dopamine. This hormonal equilibrium contributes to emotional well-being.

Emotional Resilience: Through mindfulness and self-awareness, meditation and yoga help individuals develop emotional resilience. They learn to process emotions more effectively, leading to a greater sense of emotional stability.

Spirituality and Inner Growth: Both practices have deep spiritual roots and can foster a sense of connection with something greater than oneself. This spiritual dimension allows individuals to explore their inner selves, develop a greater understanding of life's purpose, and experience personal growth.

Enhanced Respiratory Function: Breathing techniques (pranayama) used in yoga can improve lung capacity, respiratory efficiency, and overall respiratory health.

Posture Improvement: Yoga focuses on body alignment and awareness, leading to better posture and reducing the risk of musculoskeletal issues.

Weight Management: While not a substitute for a balanced diet and exercise, regular yoga practice can contribute to weight management by increasing physical activity and mindfulness around eating habits.

Self-Acceptance and Mindfulness: Both meditation and yoga encourage self-acceptance and self-compassion, promoting a more positive self-image and a non-judgmental approach to oneself and others.

Overview

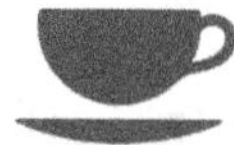

MEDITATION AND YOGA promote inner peace, mindfulness, and well-being.

Meditation is a mental practice that involves training the mind to focus and redirect thoughts. It aims to cultivate mindfulness, awareness, and a heightened state of consciousness. The primary focus of meditation is to quiet the mind, observe thoughts without judgment, and attain a deep sense of inner peace.

Yoga is a holistic practice that integrates physical postures (asanas), breath control (pranayama), meditation, and ethical principles. The primary focus of yoga is to achieve harmony between the mind, body, and spirit. While meditation is a part of yoga, yoga encompasses a broader range of practices that promote physical, mental, and spiritual well-being.

The roots of meditation can be traced back thousands of years to ancient civilizations such as India, China, and Egypt. Various forms of meditation emerged independently in different cultures, each with its own techniques and objectives. Over time, meditation evolved and spread to different parts of the world, adapting to the beliefs and practices of various societies.

Yoga also has ancient origins, dating back over 5,000 years in the Indian subcontinent. The word "yoga" is derived from the Sanskrit word "yuj," meaning to unite or yoke. Yoga originated as a spiritual discipline and philosophical system that sought to unify the individual soul with the universal consciousness. It has been transmitted through generations, with different schools of thought and styles evolving over time.

There are numerous meditation techniques, each emphasizing a unique approach to achieve mental stillness and inner awareness. Some popular meditation techniques include:

Focusing on the present moment without judgment. Cultivating feelings of love and compassion towards oneself and others. Using a mantra or sound to transcend ordinary thought patterns. Following the instructions of a guide or recorded meditation to facilitate relaxation and inner exploration.

Yoga encompasses a wide array of practices that go beyond meditation. The core practices of yoga include:

Asanas (Physical postures): Various yoga poses that improve flexibility, strength, and balance.

Pranayama (Breath control): Techniques that regulate and deepen breathing to enhance energy flow and promote relaxation.

Dhyana (Meditation): A part of yoga that involves deep concentration and contemplation.

Yamas and Niyamas (Ethical guidelines): Principles that guide ethical behavior and self-discipline.

Meditation is primarily a mental practice and does not involve specific physical postures or movements. Practitioners typically sit or lie down in a comfortable position while focusing their attention on a particular object, thought, or sensation.

Yoga incorporates physical postures (asanas) as a fundamental aspect of its practice. Different styles of yoga involve various sequences of asanas, each targeting different muscle groups and promoting flexibility, strength, and overall physical health.

Meditation can be practiced with or without a spiritual context. While it has deep spiritual roots in many traditions, meditation can also be used as a secular practice for relaxation, stress reduction, and improving focus.

Yoga, as originally conceived, is deeply rooted in spirituality and philosophy. It aims to unite the individual soul (atman) with the universal consciousness (Brahman). However, modern yoga has taken on diverse forms, and many practitioners approach it purely as a physical exercise without a spiritual dimension.

The primary purpose of meditation is to cultivate mindfulness, inner peace, and self-awareness. It aims to reduce mental chatter, alleviate stress, and gain clarity of thought. Meditation can lead to a deeper understanding of oneself and the world, fostering emotional resilience and personal growth.

The goals of yoga encompass physical, mental, and spiritual well-being. While physical fitness is a component of yoga, its ultimate aim is to achieve harmony between the mind, body, and spirit. By integrating the practices of asanas, pranayama, and meditation, yoga seeks to promote holistic health, self-realization, and spiritual growth.

Meditation can be practiced virtually anywhere and requires minimal equipment or space. It can be done in a short amount of time, making it easily accessible for individuals with busy schedules.

Depending on the style and intensity of yoga, it may require more time, space, and equipment (such as yoga mats and props). Some yoga sessions can last anywhere from 30 minutes to over an hour, making it more time-consuming compared to shorter meditation sessions.

While guided meditation sessions with instructors or recorded audio are available, meditation is often practiced as a solitary activity. Many individuals prefer self-guided meditation to explore their thoughts and emotions without external influence.

Yoga classes are typically instructor-led, especially for beginners. The presence of a yoga teacher can provide guidance on proper alignment and ensure that students perform poses safely and effectively.

Meditation has been shown to activate the parasympathetic nervous system, responsible for the body's relaxation response. This activation leads to reduced heart rate, blood pressure, and stress hormone levels.

The combination of physical movement, breath control, and meditation in yoga can have a profound effect on the autonomic nervous system, promoting both relaxation and energy balance.

Meditation is widely used for stress reduction, anxiety management, and enhancing emotional well-being. It is also employed as a complementary therapy in healthcare settings to support patients dealing with chronic pain, depression, and other medical conditions.

Yoga's diverse practices offer a wide range of benefits, including improved physical fitness, enhanced flexibility, stress reduction, and increased self-awareness. Additionally, yoga's holistic approach can foster positive changes in lifestyle, leading to better overall health and a sense of well-being.

Meditation centres on the mind and consciousness, while yoga encompasses a holistic approach that includes physical postures, breath control, meditation, and ethical principles. Each practice offers a diverse array of techniques and can be adapted to suit individual preferences and needs. Whether used independently or in tandem, meditation and yoga remain powerful tools for promoting well-being, self-awareness, and a more balanced and harmonious life.

Understanding Meditation

MEDITATION IS A TRANSFORMATIVE practice that has been cultivated and refined for millennia, deeply rooted in various religious and spiritual traditions across the world. However, in recent times, it has gained increasing popularity as a secular, non-religious practice aimed at promoting mental and emotional well-being. Understanding meditation requires delving into its origins, core principles, techniques, and the scientific evidence that supports its numerous benefits.

At its essence, meditation is a mental training technique that involves focusing one's attention and awareness to achieve a state of heightened clarity, inner calm, and self-awareness. The word "meditation" comes from the Latin word "meditatio," meaning to ponder or contemplate. In Eastern traditions, the term "meditation" generally refers to a wide range of practices that lead to heightened states of consciousness, such as dhyana in Hinduism and Buddhism. Each tradition offers various techniques, but they all share common underlying principles: concentration, mindfulness, and cultivating a non-judgmental awareness of the present moment.

Concentration meditation, also known as focused attention meditation, involves fixing one's attention on a single point of focus, such as the breath, a mantra, or an image. By continually redirecting the mind to this point of focus, practitioners learn to develop greater control over their wandering thoughts, leading to increased mental clarity and reduced distractions.

Mindfulness meditation, on the other hand, entails cultivating an open and non-reactive awareness of one's thoughts, emotions, bodily sensations, and surrounding environment. Instead of trying to block out thoughts or emotions, individuals practicing mindfulness meditation observe them without judgment or attachment. This non-judgmental stance allows for a deeper understanding of the mind's patterns and reactions, leading to enhanced emotional regulation and self-acceptance.

As meditation practices evolved over centuries, they took on distinct forms across different cultures and belief systems. For instance, in Buddhism, the Noble Eightfold Path includes "Right Mindfulness" and "Right Concentration" as essential components of the journey toward enlightenment. In contrast, Islamic tradition emphasizes meditation on the 99 Names of Allah, with the objective of deepening one's connection with the Divine.

In recent decades, numerous scientific studies have explored the effects of meditation on physical and mental health. Neuroscientific research using brain imaging technologies, such as functional magnetic resonance imaging (fMRI) and electroencephalography (EEG), has shed light on the neural mechanisms underpinning meditation's benefits.

Studies have shown that regular meditation practice can lead to structural and functional changes in the brain. One such area of interest is the anterior cingulate cortex (ACC), which plays a crucial role in attention regulation and emotional processing. Meditation has been found to increase the thickness of the ACC, leading to improved focus and emotional resilience.

Moreover, meditation appears to influence the default mode network (DMN), a brain network involved in mind-wandering and self-referential thinking. Heightened activity in the DMN is often associated with rumination and anxiety. Through meditation, individuals can reduce DMN activity, leading to decreased rumination and a greater ability to stay present in the moment.

Aside from brain changes, meditation has been linked to various physiological benefits. Studies have demonstrated that regular meditation practice can reduce blood pressure, lower cortisol levels (the stress hormone), and enhance immune system functioning. Additionally, meditation has been shown to promote better sleep and help alleviate symptoms of anxiety, depression, and post-traumatic stress disorder (PTSD).

Beyond the individual level, the benefits of meditation extend to interpersonal relationships and overall well-being. By cultivating self-awareness and emotional regulation, meditation can lead to greater empathy and compassion toward others. This, in turn, fosters healthier and more fulfilling social connections, promoting a sense of belonging and reducing feelings of loneliness.

While meditation offers numerous benefits, establishing a consistent practice can be challenging. The busy and fast-paced nature of modern life often leaves little room for introspection and self-reflection. Moreover, many beginners struggle with the misconception that meditation requires clearing the mind of all thoughts, leading to frustration when they find their minds wandering.

Patience and persistence are crucial in developing a meditation practice. Accepting that thoughts will inevitably arise during meditation and gently redirecting the focus back to the chosen point of attention is an integral part of the process. With time and practice, individuals can cultivate a more profound sense of presence and serenity.

Various meditation techniques exist to suit individual preferences and needs. Breath awareness meditation involves focusing on the sensation of breathing, which serves as an anchor to maintain concentration. Loving-kindness meditation focuses on generating feelings of compassion and goodwill toward oneself and others. Body scan meditation involves systematically bringing attention to different parts of the body, promoting relaxation and awareness of bodily sensations.

Guided meditations, where practitioners follow the instructions of a meditation teacher or audio recording, can be helpful, especially for beginners. Mindfulness-Based Stress Reduction (MBSR) and Mindfulness-Based Cognitive Therapy (MBCT) are structured programs that incorporate meditation and mindfulness practices to address specific issues like stress, anxiety, and depression.

Meditation is a versatile tool that can be adapted to various settings and contexts. Besides formal sitting meditation, mindfulness can be integrated into daily activities, such as eating, walking, or even washing dishes. Engaging in such activities with full awareness brings a sense of grounded-ness and appreciation for the simple moments of life.

Moreover, many businesses and organizations have started incorporating mindfulness practices into their workplaces to improve employee well-being and productivity. Mindful leadership, which involves making decisions with greater clarity and empathy, has become a sought-after skill for effective leaders.

In conclusion, meditation is a profound and multifaceted practice that offers a path to greater self-awareness, emotional well-being, and spiritual growth. Its evolution across various traditions and cultures has led to a wide range of meditation techniques, each with unique approaches and goals. Modern scientific research has validated many of the claimed benefits of meditation, highlighting its transformative effects on the brain, body, and overall health.

However, it is essential to recognize that meditation is not a quick fix or a one-size-fits-all solution. Like any skill, it requires consistent effort and patience to cultivate. By embracing meditation as a journey of self-discovery and inner exploration, individuals can unlock its potential for personal growth and profound transformation. Whether seeking stress relief, emotional balance, or spiritual awakening, the practice of meditation holds the promise of a more fulfilling and meaningful life.

The importance of being present in the moment and observing thoughts without judgment

MEDITATION IS A PROFOUND practice that holds the potential to unlock inner peace, self-awareness, and a deeper connection with the present moment. As individuals' journey through the art of meditation, they embark on a path of self-discovery and transformation. Although meditation encompasses various techniques and traditions, the core steps remain consistent across different practices. Here, we delve into these fundamental steps that guide practitioners in their quest for inner stillness and heightened consciousness.

Find a Comfortable Posture

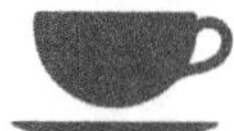

THE FIRST STEP IN MEDITATION involves finding a comfortable posture that supports both alertness and relaxation. Traditionally, meditation is practiced in a seated position, either on the floor or a cushion, with legs crossed in a lotus or half-lotus position. However, practitioners can also sit on a chair or use any other comfortable sitting position that keeps the spine straight and aligned. The hands may rest on the lap, with palms facing upward or downward, forming a gentle mudra. The shoulders are relaxed, and the chin is slightly tucked in to maintain a sense of balance and openness.

Settle into the Present Moment

WITH THE PHYSICAL POSTURE established, the next step involves grounding oneself in the present moment. Practitioners take a few deep breaths, tuning into the sensations of the body and the rhythm of the breath. By anchoring attention to the present, one begins to let go of distractions and mental chatter, gradually entering a state of relaxed awareness.

Focus on the Breath

ONE OF THE MOST COMMON meditation techniques involves focusing on the breath. As practitioners settle into the present moment, they direct their attention to the natural flow of the breath—feeling the coolness of the inhalation and the warmth of the exhalation. Observing the breath serves as an anchor to prevent the mind from wandering and brings a sense of centeredness to the practice.

Observe Thoughts Without Judgment

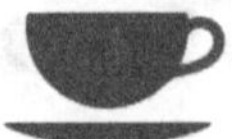

AS PRACTITIONERS CONCENTRATE on the breath, thoughts inevitably arise. The key to this step lies in observing these thoughts without judgment or attachment. Rather than getting entangled in the thought stream, practitioners gently bring their attention back to the breath each time the mind wanders. This process of non-judgmental observation cultivates mindfulness—a state of awareness without reactivity or emotional entanglement.

Cultivate Non-Attachment

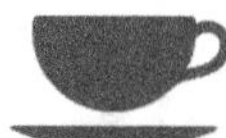

BUILDING UPON THE PREVIOUS step, meditation encourages practitioners to cultivate non-attachment to thoughts, emotions, and sensations that arise during the practice. By recognizing that thoughts are transient mental events and not inherent aspects of the self, individuals develop a sense of detachment from their cognitive processes. This non-attachment allows for greater mental clarity and emotional equanimity.

Embrace Acceptance and Compassion

MEDITATION IS NOT ABOUT eliminating thoughts or emotions but rather embracing them with acceptance and compassion. As practitioners observe their inner experiences without judgment, they extend kindness and understanding to themselves. This self-compassion creates a safe space for emotional healing and personal growth, fostering a deeper connection with one's inner world.

Cultivate Loving-Kindness (Metta)

IN ADDITION TO SELF-compassion, many meditation practices incorporate the cultivation of loving-kindness (Metta) toward oneself and others. Metta meditation involves silently repeating positive affirmations or phrases, such as "May I be happy, may I be healthy, may I live with ease." Gradually, these well-wishes are extended to loved ones, neutral individuals, and even challenging people. This practice helps in nurturing empathy and interconnectedness with all beings.

Focus on a Specific Object

APART FROM THE BREATH, meditation can involve focusing attention on a specific object or sensation. This object of focus could be a candle flame, a mantra, a sound, or a visual image. By honing attention on a singular point, practitioners cultivate concentration and single-pointed awareness, which are foundational to deeper meditative states.

Explore Body Scan Meditation

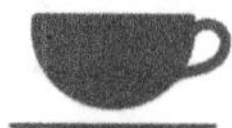

BODY SCAN MEDITATION is another valuable technique where attention is systematically directed to different parts of the body. Practitioners explore bodily sensations with open curiosity and non-judgmental awareness. This practice enhances somatic awareness and relaxation, promoting a profound sense of being in tune with the physical self.

Engage in Walking Meditation

MEDITATION IS NOT CONFINED to sitting practices alone; it can be integrated into daily activities, including walking. Walking meditation involves slow, deliberate steps with full awareness of each movement. Practitioners focus on the sensations in their feet and legs as they lift, move, and place each foot. Walking meditation nurtures a sense of mindfulness in motion, allowing individuals to connect with the environment and their bodies in a unique way.

Develop Gratitude

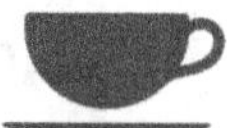

GRATITUDE MEDITATION involves reflecting on the positive aspects of life and cultivating a sense of gratitude for them. By acknowledging and appreciating the blessings and abundance in one's life, practitioners shift their focus from lack to abundance, fostering a greater sense of contentment and joy.

Cultivate Equanimity

EQUANIMITY IS THE ABILITY to maintain composure and balance amidst life's ups and downs. Meditation supports the development of equanimity by teaching practitioners to embrace impermanence and uncertainty with acceptance. This allows individuals to navigate the waves of life's challenges and joys with grace and resilience.

Practice Mindful Eating

MINDFUL EATING IS AN invitation to savour each bite of food with full presence and appreciation. By engaging the senses and observing the tastes, textures, and aromas of the meal, individuals cultivate a deeper connection with the nourishment they receive. Mindful eating promotes healthier eating habits and a greater sense of gratitude for the sustenance that nourishes the body.

Cultivate Patience and Persistence

MEDITATION IS A GRADUAL journey that requires patience and persistence. The mind's propensity to wander or become restless is entirely normal, especially for beginners. Instead of becoming discouraged, practitioners are encouraged to approach meditation with a gentle determination, understanding that progress unfolds over time.

Transcendental Meditation (TM)

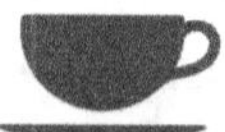

FROM THE ANCIENT WISDOM of Vedic traditions emerges Transcendental Meditation (TM), a technique that invites practitioners to access a state of transcendent consciousness—a realm beyond ordinary awareness. Practitioners use a silent, personal mantra, gently repeating it during meditation, which allows the mind to effortlessly transcend the surface level of thoughts and enter into a state of deep relaxation and inner peace.

Zen Meditation (Zazen)

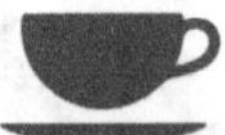

STEEPED IN ZEN BUDDHISM, Zazen is a minimalist and profound form of meditation that emphasizes seated meditation (seiza). Practitioners focus on their breath or engage in "Koan" contemplation— a paradoxical question or statement— to transcend dualistic thinking. In this practice, the mind is invited to rest in the "suchness" of the present moment, beyond conceptualization or judgment.

Vipassana Meditation

ROOTED IN THE TEACHINGS of the Buddha, Vipassana meditation (insight meditation) is an ancient technique that delves into the impermanent and ever-changing nature of reality. Practitioners observe bodily sensations, thoughts, and emotions with unwavering attention, developing profound insight into the interconnectedness of all phenomena and the nature of suffering and liberation.

Chakra Meditation

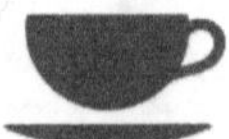

WITHIN THE RICH TAPESTRY of yogic traditions, Chakra meditation arises as a transformative practice that focuses on the seven main energy centres (chakras) in the body. Through visualization, chanting, or energy-awareness techniques, practitioners seek to cleanse, balance, and activate these energy centres, fostering harmony and alignment in the physical, emotional, and spiritual dimensions.

Guided Visualization

GUIDED VISUALIZATION is a meditative technique that employs mental imagery to evoke specific experiences or sensations. With the guidance of a teacher or a recorded audio, practitioners embark on inner journeys, imagining peaceful settings, personal goals, or transformative experiences. This technique helps foster relaxation, focus, and the power of the mind to manifest intentions.

Body Scan Meditation

A MEDITATIVE JOURNEY of somatic awareness, body scan meditation invites practitioners to explore the body with a gentle and non-judgmental gaze. Starting from the toes and gradually moving upward, practitioners observe bodily sensations, tensions, and emotions, cultivating a deep sense of presence and relaxation.

Sound Bath Meditation

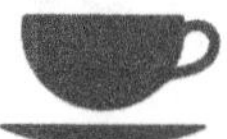

IN THE REALM OF SOUND, lies a meditative practice known as sound bath meditation, where the vibrations of various instruments, such as singing bowls, gongs, or chimes, bathe practitioners in a sea of harmonic frequencies. The ethereal sounds lead to a state of deep relaxation and inner stillness, guiding practitioners into altered states of consciousness and profound inner healing.

Body-Oriented Meditation (e.g., Yoga, Tai Chi, Qigong):

BEYOND THE TRADITIONAL seated practices, body-oriented meditation techniques, such as Yoga, Tai Chi, and Qigong, offer a holistic and integrated approach to meditation. Combining breathwork, movement, and mindfulness, these practices harmonize the body, mind, and spirit, fostering physical strength, flexibility, and mental clarity.

Compassion Meditation (Tonglen)

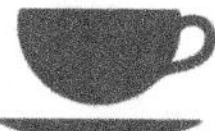

AN ANCIENT TIBETAN practice, Tonglen meditation, encapsulates the essence of compassion. In this practice, practitioners breathe in the suffering of others, transmuting it into healing and compassion, and breathe out loving-kindness and relief. This powerful technique opens the heart to embrace the pain of the world with fearless love and empathy.

Body-Observation Meditation
(Vipassana)

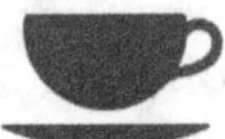

A VARIANT OF VIPASSANA meditation, body-observation meditation invites practitioners to explore the sensations and experiences within the body, transcending the duality between self and body. This practice fosters a profound sense of unity and connection with the physical vessel that houses the soul.

Nada Yoga (Sound Yoga)

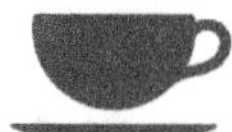

WITHIN THE DOMAIN OF yoga, Nada Yoga—a practice that harmonizes the mind through sound—rings like a celestial melody. Practitioners turn inward, focusing on inner sounds and vibrations, perceiving the soundless sound (Anahata Nada) that resonates with the rhythm of the cosmos, guiding them into a state of meditative bliss.

Exercise and Physical Activity

EMBARKING ON THE PATH of healing, exercise and physical activity emerge as allies in the quest for well-being. Engaging in regular exercise releases endorphins, the brain's natural mood-enhancing chemicals, promoting a sense of euphoria and reducing stress. Whether through cardio workouts, yoga, or nature walks, physical activity provides an outlet for emotional release, a respite from daily stressors, and a boost to self-confidence.

Social Support and Connection

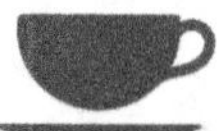

IN THE TAPESTRY OF healing, social support and connection are threads of essential significance. Sharing the burdens of stress, anxiety, and depression with empathetic friends, family, or support groups creates a safety net of understanding and compassion. Genuine connections foster a sense of belonging, reduce feelings of isolation, and create a space where individuals can openly share their emotions and experiences, fostering healing and growth.

Cognitive Behavioral Therapy (CBT)

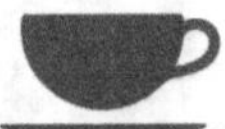

WITHIN THE REALM OF therapeutic approaches, Cognitive Behavioral Therapy (CBT) stands as a guiding light. CBT is a well-established, evidence-based practice that empowers individuals to identify negative thought patterns and replace them with healthier and more adaptive thoughts. By reframing perceptions and challenging cognitive distortions, individuals learn coping strategies to navigate stressors and lessen the impact of anxiety and depression.

Self-Compassion and Acceptance

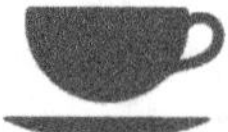

AS SEEKERS EMBRACE the path of healing, the practice of self-compassion and self-acceptance becomes a soothing balm for emotional wounds. Embracing imperfections, treating oneself with kindness, and releasing the shackles of self-criticism fosters a profound sense of inner peace. By being gentle with oneself and acknowledging that struggles are a natural part of the human experience, individuals can find the strength to overcome challenges with resilience and grace.

Nature and Ecotherapy

AMIDST THE HUSTLE AND bustle of modern life, nature emerges as a sanctuary for restoration and healing. Ecotherapy, or nature-based therapy, advocates spending time in natural settings to alleviate stress and improve mental well-being. The sights, sounds, and smells of nature connect individuals with the present moment, offering a sense of tranquillity and awe that lessens the grip of anxiety and depression.

Creative Expression

WITHIN THE REALM OF art and creative expression, the soul finds respite from the tumult of stress, anxiety, and depression. Engaging in creative pursuits such as painting, music, dance, or writing unlocks the flow of emotions, channelling them into a cathartic and empowering medium. Creativity becomes a pathway to inner transformation, fostering a sense of accomplishment and joy.

Integrate Meditation into Daily Life

AS THE FORMAL PRACTICE of meditation becomes an integral part of one's routine, the final step involves integrating mindfulness into daily life. This entails bringing the awareness cultivated during meditation into everyday activities, interactions, and moments. By living mindfully, individuals enrich their experience of life, fostering a profound sense of interconnectedness and authenticity.

The meditation's steps form a tapestry of inner exploration, fostering self-awareness, compassion, and equanimity. Through the practice of meditation, individuals transcend the limitations of the ego, embracing the vastness of their inner landscapes and the boundless unity that connects all beings. As they embark on this transformative journey, they unlock the door to profound serenity, attaining a timeless sanctuary of presence and a renewed appreciation for the art of simply being.

Reduce stress, anxiety, and depression

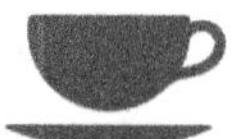

REDUCING STRESS, ANXIETY, and depression is a vital endeavour that empowers individuals to reclaim their emotional well-being and nurture a harmonious mind-body connection. In the modern world, where relentless demands and constant stimuli abound, the quest to alleviate these psychological burdens becomes ever more crucial. Fortunately, a myriad of evidence-based approaches, spanning from lifestyle changes to therapeutic interventions, offers a rich tapestry of tools to embark on this transformative journey. By cultivating self-awareness, fostering resilience, and embracing a holistic perspective, individuals can forge a path towards a more serene and emotionally balanced existence.

At the heart of stress reduction lies the practice of mindfulness a timeless technique that has garnered increasing attention in contemporary psychology and well-being. Mindfulness, rooted in ancient contemplative traditions, invites individuals to embrace the present moment with non-judgmental awareness. Through mindful practices such as meditation, deep breathing, and body scans, individuals learn to detach from the harried thoughts of the past and the anxieties of the future. By nurturing a profound connection with the here and now, they gain the power to interrupt the cascade of stress responses and foster a calm and centred state of mind.

Moreover, mindfulness-based interventions, such as Mindfulness-Based Stress Reduction (MBSR) and Mindfulness-Based Cognitive Therapy (MBCT), have demonstrated significant efficacy in reducing stress, anxiety, and depression. By combining mindfulness practices with cognitive-behavioural techniques, these interventions equip individuals with the tools to identify and transform negative thought patterns, cultivate self-compassion, and promote emotional regulation. As a result, practitioners become more adept at navigating life's challenges with resilience and a newfound sense of peace.

Beyond mindfulness, engaging in regular physical exercise emerges as a potent ally in reducing stress, anxiety, and depression. Exercise, whether it be aerobic activities, yoga, or tai chi, stimulates the release of endorphins—the brain's natural feel-good chemicals. These endorphins act as a buffer against stress, elevating mood and promoting a sense of well-being. Moreover, exercise fosters a deeper mind-body connection, allowing individuals to release physical tension and emotional stress, thus facilitating a holistic approach to stress reduction.

Another powerful avenue for reducing stress, anxiety, and depression lies in nurturing meaningful social connections. Human beings are inherently social creatures, and the quality of our relationships profoundly impacts our emotional health. Engaging in positive social interactions, seeking support from loved ones, and participating in community activities fosters a sense of belonging and safety. These supportive networks act as a buffer against stress and promote emotional resilience, offering solace during times of difficulty.

In the therapeutic realm, Cognitive-Behavioural Therapy (CBT) emerges as a well-established and effective approach for addressing stress, anxiety, and depression. CBT operates on the premise that our thoughts, emotions, and behaviours are interconnected. By identifying and challenging negative thought patterns and adopting healthier cognitive strategies, individuals can reframe their perceptions of stressors and promote emotional well-being. CBT equips individuals with practical coping skills, empowering them to navigate stressful situations with greater ease and confidence.

Furthermore, addressing lifestyle factors can have a profound impact on stress reduction. Sleep plays a critical role in emotional regulation, and chronic sleep deprivation can exacerbate stress, anxiety, and depression. Prioritizing restful sleep by establishing consistent sleep routines, creating a relaxing bedtime environment, and managing screen time before sleep can significantly enhance well-being. Additionally, practicing good nutrition, staying hydrated, and avoiding excessive consumption of stimulants like caffeine and alcohol contribute to emotional balance and stress management.

In some cases, stress, anxiety, and depression may require professional intervention, especially when symptoms persist or significantly impact daily functioning. Mental health professionals, such as psychologists, counsellors, and psychiatrists, offer specialized support and guidance in addressing these challenges. Through psychotherapy, individuals gain a safe space to explore underlying emotional issues, process trauma, and develop coping strategies tailored to their unique needs. Medication may also be prescribed by a psychiatrist to manage symptoms and support the healing process, particularly in cases of severe or persistent anxiety and depression.

As part of a comprehensive approach, incorporating relaxation techniques can provide valuable relief from stress, anxiety, and depression. Practices such as progressive muscle relaxation, guided imagery, and deep breathing exercises offer a soothing respite from the demands of daily life. Engaging in hobbies, creative activities, or spending time in nature can further promote relaxation and emotional rejuvenation, allowing individuals to find moments of joy amidst life's challenges.

Moreover, practicing self-compassion plays an integral role in reducing stress, anxiety, and depression. Often, individuals are their harshest critics, holding themselves to unrealistic standards and berating themselves for perceived shortcomings. By offering themselves the same kindness and understanding they would extend to a friend, individuals foster emotional resilience and promote a positive relationship with themselves.

For some, engaging in spiritual or contemplative practices can provide a profound sense of meaning and purpose, guiding them through difficult times. Prayer, meditation, or connecting with one's sense of spirituality can serve as sources of solace and strength, encouraging individuals to view their struggles from a broader perspective.

Improve focus and concentration

IMPROVING FOCUS AND concentration through meditation is a transformative journey that empowers individuals to harness the power of their minds and cultivate a profound sense of presence and clarity. In the ever-changing and fast-paced world we live in, distractions abound, making it challenging to stay focused on tasks and activities that demand our attention. As seekers embark on this profound path, they weave together the threads of mindfulness, meditation, and self-awareness, creating a tapestry of mental resilience and unwavering focus. From the depths of breath-centred practices to the heights of transcendental meditation, each meditation technique intertwines to cultivate a focused and concentrated mind, illuminating the path towards enhanced productivity, creativity, and overall well-being.

Mindfulness Meditation: At the heart of improving focus and concentration lies mindfulness meditation—an ancient practice rooted in Buddhist traditions. Mindfulness involves paying non-judgmental attention to the present moment, observing thoughts, emotions, and sensations without attachment or aversion. Through regular mindfulness practice, individuals develop the ability to stay fully engaged in the task at hand, letting go of distractions and increasing their cognitive control.

Concentration Meditation (Samatha): Concentration meditation, also known as Samatha, involves focusing the mind on a single point of attention, such as the breath, a mantra, or a visual object. By repeatedly bringing the mind back to the chosen focal point, practitioners strengthen their mental focus and develop the capacity to sustain attention for extended periods.

Open Monitoring Meditation: Open monitoring meditation involves observing thoughts and sensations as they arise without getting caught up in them. By maintaining a detached and non-reactive awareness, individuals cultivate mental clarity and a heightened ability to sustain attention.

Benefits of Meditation

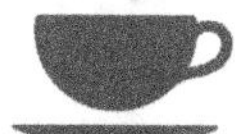

MEDITATION, AN ANCIENT practice that has stood the test of time, unveils a profound tapestry of physical benefits that envelop the body in a cloak of healing and well-being. Beyond its reputation for calming the mind and nurturing inner peace, meditation serves as a powerful elixir, harmonizing the mind-body connection and bestowing a myriad of physical rewards. As seekers embark on this transformative journey, they unravel the intertwined threads of mindfulness, relaxation, and stress reduction, revealing a canvas of improved physical health, enhanced immune function, and heightened vitality. From the depths of reduced inflammation to the heights of lowered blood pressure, each thread weaves together to create a fabric of holistic health, illuminating the path towards a life of vibrancy, longevity, and radiant well-being.

Stress Reduction and Cortisol Regulation: At the core of meditation's physical benefits lies its ability to reduce stress and regulate cortisol—the body's primary stress hormone. As individuals practice meditation, they activate the relaxation response, triggering a cascade of physiological changes that lower cortisol levels. By mitigating the harmful effects of chronic stress, meditation supports overall well-being and reduces the risk of stress-related health issues.

Enhanced Immune Function: Within the realm of immune health, meditation emerges as a powerful ally. Studies have shown that regular meditation strengthens the immune system, increasing the production of immune cells and antibodies. A robust immune system better equips the body to defend against infections, illnesses, and chronic diseases, fostering optimal health and vitality.

Lowered Blood Pressure: In the sanctuary of heart health, meditation stands as a pillar of support. Meditation has been linked to reduced blood pressure, promoting cardiovascular well-being and reducing the risk of heart disease. By calming the sympathetic nervous system—the "fight or flight" response—meditation nurtures a state of relaxation that supports healthy blood pressure levels.

Improved Heart Health: Beyond lowering blood pressure, meditation enriches heart health through other mechanisms. Studies have demonstrated that meditation reduces cholesterol levels, lowers triglycerides, and improves arterial function. By supporting heart health, meditation becomes a key player in preventing heart disease and promoting longevity.

Enhanced Respiratory Function: In the realm of respiratory health, meditation becomes a source of nourishment. By encouraging mindful breathing and relaxation, meditation optimizes lung capacity and respiratory function. Individuals with respiratory conditions, such as asthma, may experience relief through meditation's calming effects on the respiratory system.

Reduced Inflammation: Chronic inflammation lies at the root of numerous health conditions, from arthritis to cardiovascular disease. Meditation's anti-inflammatory effects have been scientifically documented, as it suppresses the expression of genes associated with inflammation. By reducing inflammation, meditation becomes a potent tool in preventing and managing inflammatory-related diseases.

Pain Management: Meditation unfolds as a balm for the body, offering relief from physical pain and discomfort. Studies have shown that meditation activates brain regions involved in pain modulation, reducing the perception of pain and enhancing pain tolerance. Meditation-based pain management can complement conventional treatments, providing individuals with a holistic approach to pain relief.

Improved Sleep Quality: Within the sanctuary of restful sleep, meditation emerges as a guiding light. Regular meditation practices have been linked to improved sleep quality, reduced insomnia, and enhanced overall sleep duration. By calming the mind and promoting relaxation, meditation fosters a peaceful transition into restorative slumber.

Hormonal Balance: The endocrine system, responsible for hormone production and regulation, finds balance and harmony through meditation. Studies indicate that meditation modulates hormonal activity, leading to improved hormonal balance and overall well-being. Balanced hormones contribute to better mood, energy levels, and reproductive health.

Digestive Health: Amidst the intricacies of the digestive system, meditation offers a sanctuary of support. Stress and anxiety can disrupt digestion, leading to digestive discomfort and conditions like irritable bowel syndrome (IBS). Through its stress-reducing effects, meditation promotes healthy digestion and alleviates gastrointestinal disturbances.

Weight Management: In the realm of body weight, meditation becomes a gentle guide. By fostering self-awareness and mindfulness around eating habits, meditation supports healthy eating behaviours and conscious food choices. Additionally, meditation reduces stress, which can contribute to emotional eating and weight gain.

Slowed Cellular Aging: Within the fabric of longevity, meditation unveils its anti-aging properties. Telomeres—the protective caps at the ends of chromosomes—are markers of cellular aging. Regular meditation has been associated with longer telomeres, indicating slower cellular aging and potential longevity benefits.

Enhanced Cognitive Function: The mind's vitality finds expression through meditation's impact on cognitive function. Studies have shown that meditation improves memory, attention, and cognitive flexibility. By fostering a focused and clear mind, meditation enhances cognitive abilities and mental acuity.

Regulation of Autonomic Nervous System: The autonomic nervous system, responsible for regulating involuntary bodily functions, finds balance through meditation. By activating the parasympathetic nervous system, the "rest and digest" response meditation counteracts the stress-induced activation of the sympathetic nervous system, promoting overall physiological balance.

Strengthened Mind-Body Connection: In the realm of mind-body integration, meditation emerges as a guiding force. By cultivating self-awareness and a deep connection with the present moment, meditation nurtures a harmonious relationship between the mind and body. This heightened mind-body connection empowers individuals to better understand their physical needs and respond to them with care and intuition.

The physical benefits of meditation unfold as a symphony of healing and well-being. As seekers embrace the transformative journey of meditation, they unravel the tapestry of stress reduction, enhanced immune function, and improved heart health. Through meditation's calming effects on the mind and body, they experience lowered blood pressure, reduced inflammation, and a deeper connection with their physical being. The interplay of mindfulness and relaxation fosters a profound state of rest and rejuvenation, supporting improved sleep quality and pain management. In the realm of hormonal balance and digestive health, meditation's therapeutic embrace nurtures holistic well-being. As individuals weave the threads of meditation into the fabric of their lives, they find themselves enveloped in a cloak of vibrant health, radiating vitality, and embodying the boundless potential of the mind-body connection. In the sanctuary of meditation, they discover the keys to unlock the treasures of physical health, enriching their lives with longevity, resilience, and the gift of holistic well-being.

The Essentials of Yoga

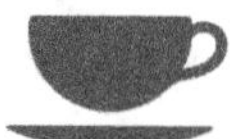

YOGA, A TIMELESS PRACTICE that unites body, mind, and spirit, unveils a profound tapestry of essentials that embody its transformative power. Rooted in ancient Indian traditions, yoga has transcended time and cultural boundaries to become a global phenomenon embraced by millions. As seekers embark on this transformative journey, they unravel the intertwined threads of physical postures (asanas), breath control (pranayama), and meditation (dhyana), revealing a canvas of holistic well-being, inner harmony, and self-discovery. From the depths of flexibility and strength to the heights of mental clarity and spiritual awakening, each thread weaves together to create a fabric of balance, vitality, and profound consciousness, illuminating the path towards a life of radiance, serenity, and self-awareness.

Asanas (Physical Postures): At the core of yoga's essentials lies the practice of asanas—physical postures that promote flexibility, strength, and balance. As individuals flow through a diverse array of poses, they cultivate awareness of their bodies, fostering a deeper connection with their physical selves. Asanas not only enhance physical fitness but also promote mental focus and relaxation, paving the way for a more harmonious integration of body and mind.

Pranayama (Breath Control): Within the realm of breath, pranayama emerges as a vital aspect of yoga. Prana, the life force energy, is harnessed and regulated through various breathing techniques. By consciously controlling the breath, practitioners achieve a state of calmness, purify their energy channels, and access deeper levels of consciousness. Pranayama serves as a bridge between the physical and spiritual dimensions of yoga, nurturing the mind-body connection.

Meditation (Dhyana): Meditation stands as a pillar of yoga's essentials, inviting individuals to journey within and explore the realms of their inner landscape. Through meditation, practitioners cultivate mindfulness, focus, and self-awareness. This transformative practice leads to mental clarity, emotional balance, and a deeper understanding of the self. Meditation unveils the wisdom that lies within, guiding individuals towards spiritual growth and self-discovery.

Yoga Philosophy and Ethics: Beyond the physical and mental dimensions, yoga's foundation rests on a rich philosophy and ethical principles that guide practitioners towards virtuous living. The eight-fold path of yoga, as described by Patanjali in the Yoga Sutras, includes principles such as non-violence (ahimsa), truthfulness (satya), and contentment (santosha). These principles offer a compass for conscious living and foster a harmonious relationship with oneself, others, and the world.

Mind-Body Connection: In the sanctuary of the mind-body connection, yoga becomes a guiding force. The practice of yoga unites breath, movement, and awareness, nurturing a profound connection between the physical and mental aspects of the self. Through asanas and pranayama, practitioners cultivate mindfulness and present-moment awareness, deepening the integration of mind and body.

Flexibility and Strength: Within the realm of physical fitness, yoga serves as an exceptional means to improve flexibility and strength. Asanas require a combination of stretching and muscle engagement, enhancing joint mobility and muscular endurance. Regular yoga practice promotes functional movement, reducing the risk of injuries and enhancing overall physical performance.

Stress Reduction and Relaxation: In the fabric of stress reduction, yoga emerges as a sanctuary of calmness and relaxation. The practice of asanas, pranayama, and meditation triggers the relaxation response, reducing stress hormones and calming the nervous system. This state of relaxation fosters mental clarity, emotional stability, and a sense of inner peace amidst life's challenges.

Improved Posture and Body Alignment: The art of body alignment unfolds within the realm of yoga, promoting improved posture and spinal health. As individuals practice asanas mindfully, they align their bodies, correcting postural imbalances and supporting the natural curvature of the spine. Enhanced body alignment fosters optimal physical function and reduces the risk of musculoskeletal issues.

Increased Energy and Vitality: Amidst the intricacies of energy flow, yoga becomes a source of vitality and rejuvenation. The practice of pranayama and asanas optimizes the flow of prana throughout the body, invigorating the entire system. This increased energy and vitality translate into improved mental focus, enhanced physical performance, and a vibrant zest for life.

Emotional Regulation and Resilience: Within the sanctuary of emotional well-being, yoga emerges as a nurturing force. The practice of yoga cultivates emotional intelligence, enabling individuals to observe and regulate their emotions with compassion and mindfulness. This emotional resilience empowers practitioners to navigate life's ups and downs with grace and equanimity.

Immune System Support: In the realm of immune health, yoga unveils its supportive nature. The practice of asanas, pranayama, and meditation enhances immune function by reducing stress, promoting relaxation, and balancing the body's energy flow. A strengthened immune system contributes to overall health and the body's ability to ward off illnesses.

Better Sleep Quality: Within the tapestry of restful sleep, yoga becomes a gentle lullaby. The practice of yoga fosters relaxation and a calm mind, setting the stage for restorative sleep. As individuals embrace mindfulness and release tension through asanas, they experience improved sleep quality and wake up feeling refreshed and rejuvenated.

Inner Awareness and Self-Discovery: Meditation unfolds as a portal to inner awareness and self-discovery within the realm of yoga. By turning the gaze inward and observing the mind's fluctuations, practitioners gain insights into their thought patterns, beliefs, and emotions. This journey of self-discovery leads to greater self-understanding and personal growth.

Detoxification and Cleansing: In the realm of physical purification, yoga emerges as a cleansing ritual. Asanas and pranayama stimulate blood circulation, lymphatic drainage, and organ function, facilitating the body's natural detoxification processes. This cleansing effect rejuvenates the body's systems and supports overall vitality.

Spiritual Awakening and Connection: Beyond the physical and mental dimensions, yoga unfolds as a pathway to spiritual awakening and connection. As individuals deepen their meditation practice, they tap into the infinite wellspring of consciousness within. This profound connection with the inner self and the universal consciousness leads to spiritual growth and a sense of oneness with all of creation.

The essentials of yoga create a tapestry of holistic well-being, radiance, and self-awareness. As seekers embrace the transformative journey of yoga, they unravel the interconnected threads of asanas, pranayama, and meditation, experiencing improved physical health, mental clarity, and emotional balance. Through the practice of yoga, they harmonize the mind-body connection, cultivating flexibility, strength, and inner harmony. The philosophy and ethics of yoga guide them towards virtuous living and a deeper understanding of the self. As they embrace the art of body alignment and emotional resilience, they uncover the keys to improved posture, increased energy, and emotional well-being. In the sanctuary of yoga, they discover the power to awaken the spirit, embark on a journey of self-discovery, and connect with the profound essence of existence. In this sacred journey, they illuminate the path towards a life of vitality, serenity, and profound consciousness, weaving together the essentials of yoga into the fabric of their lives, enriching every aspect of their being. In short meditation is related to the control of the mind and yoga is related to the control of the body.

Early yogic practices found in the Vedas and Upanishads

EARLY YOGIC PRACTICES found in the Vedas and Upanishads trace the roots of this ancient tradition back to the dawn of human civilization, where seekers and sages delved into the depths of self-discovery and spiritual awakening. The Vedas, a collection of sacred texts dating back to around 1500 BCE, and the Upanishads, philosophical treatises composed between 800 and 200 BCE, offer glimpses into the early stages of yogic knowledge and practices. These ancient scriptures serve as a sacred repository of wisdom, illuminating the essence of early yogic principles, rituals, and the quest for self-realization.

Rigveda: The Earliest Mentions of Yoga: The Rigveda, the oldest of the four Vedas, is a collection of hymns and sacred verses dating back to around 1500 BCE. Within its verses, one can find the earliest mentions of yogic concepts. The Rigveda acknowledges the importance of spiritual practices, including meditation and contemplation, as a means to connect with the divine and attain higher states of consciousness.

Atharvaveda: The Science of Healing: The Atharvaveda, another Vedic text, is distinct for its focus on practical knowledge, including healing techniques and rituals. While not explicitly focused on yoga as it is known today, the Atharvaveda contains hymns and mantras used for healing, purification, and well-being, setting the stage for the holistic approach that yoga would later embody.

Yajurveda: Rituals and Sacrifices: The Yajurveda contains verses related to rituals and sacrifices performed by Vedic priests. While it may not directly address the physical and meditative aspects of yoga, these rituals laid the foundation for later practices that incorporated physical postures and spiritual disciplines.

Samaveda: The Chants and Melodies of Yoga: The Samaveda focuses on chants and melodies used during Vedic rituals and ceremonies. These chants served to evoke a sense of devotion and reverence, foreshadowing the power of sound (mantra) as a tool for focusing the mind and deepening spiritual practices in later yogic traditions.

Early Upanishads: The Philosophy of Self-Realization: The Upanishads, composed between 800 and 200 BCE, form the philosophical portion of the Vedic literature. They delve into the nature of reality, the self (Atman), and the ultimate truth (Brahman). The Upanishads introduce the concept of self-realization, emphasizing the importance of introspection and meditation to uncover the true nature of the self.

The Bhagavad Gita: Yoga as a Path to Liberation: The Bhagavad Gita, a sacred text within the Indian epic Mahabharata, presents a profound dialogue between the warrior Arjuna and Lord Krishna. It explores the concept of dharma (righteous duty) and introduces various paths of yoga, including Karma Yoga (the yoga of selfless action), Bhakti Yoga (the yoga of devotion), and Jnana Yoga (the yoga of knowledge). The Bhagavad Gita emphasizes the importance of inner discipline and self-realization on the path to liberation.

Patanjali's Yoga Sutras: The Classical Systematization of Yoga: Composed around the 2nd century BCE, Patanjali's Yoga Sutras serve as a seminal work that systematizes the philosophy and practices of yoga. In this foundational text, Patanjali outlines the Eight Limbs of Yoga, offering a comprehensive framework for spiritual growth, self-discipline, and the attainment of Samadhi (a state of profound meditation and union with the divine).

Hatha Yoga Pradipika: The Ancient Guide to Hatha Yoga

THE HATHA YOGA PRADIPIKA, written in the 15th century CE by Swami Svatmarama, is a significant text that focuses on Hatha Yoga, the branch of yoga that emphasizes physical postures (asanas) and breath control (pranayama). This text provides instructions on various asanas, purification practices (shatkarmas), and energy channeling techniques (bandhas) to awaken the Kundalini energy and facilitate spiritual awakening.

Gheranda Samhita: The Yoga Manual of Gheranda

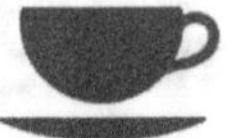

THE GHERANDA SAMHITA, composed around the 17th century CE, is another essential text of Hatha Yoga. It delves into various physical postures, breathing practices, and meditation techniques. The Gheranda Samhita emphasizes the importance of self-discipline, dedication, and commitment to the path of yoga.

Shiva Samhita: The Teachings of Lord Shiva

THE SHIVA SAMHITA, believed to be written around the 17th century CE, is a text attributed to Lord Shiva himself. It elaborates on various aspects of yoga, including asanas, pranayama, meditation, and Kundalini awakening. The Shiva Samhita also discusses the importance of a qualified teacher (guru) and the significance of devotion on the yogic path.

Tantric Yoga: The Union of Opposites

TANTRIC YOGA, WHICH emerged around the 5th century CE, emphasizes the union of opposites and the transformation of energy to attain spiritual liberation. Tantric practices integrate elements of Hatha Yoga, Kundalini Yoga, and mantra recitation to channel energy (prana) and awaken higher consciousness.

Yoga in Buddhism: The Path to Enlightenment

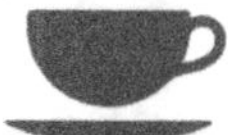

YOGA ALSO FOUND ITS way into Buddhist traditions, where it was integrated into the practices of meditation and mindfulness. In Buddhist traditions, yoga served as a path to liberation and enlightenment, aligning with the Buddha's teachings on the Four Noble Truths and the Eightfold Path.

In conclusion, early yogic practices found in the Vedas and Upanishads offer a glimpse into the rich tapestry of wisdom and self-realization that defines the essence of yoga. From the early mentions of meditation and contemplation in the Rigveda to the philosophical inquiries of the Upanishads, these ancient texts lay the groundwork for the spiritual journey of yoga. Over time, yoga evolved and branched into various traditions, including Hatha Yoga, Karma Yoga, Bhakti Yoga, Jnana Yoga, and Tantra. Today, the legacy of these early yogic practices continues to resonate, as millions of practitioners around the world embark on the transformative journey of yoga, seeking inner peace, self-discovery, and union with the divine. In the sanctuary of yoga, seekers find solace, illumination, and a profound connection with the eternal wisdom that has guided humanity on its quest for self-realization for millennia.

The Yoga Sutras and the eight limbs of yoga

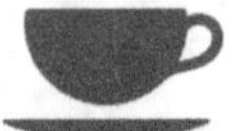

THE YOGA SUTRAS, ATTRIBUTED to the sage Patanjali, stand as a timeless and profound masterpiece that illuminates the path of yoga and unveils the essence of self-realization. Composed around the 2nd century BCE, these ancient aphorisms encapsulate the wisdom, practices, and philosophy of yoga, providing seekers with a comprehensive guide to inner transformation and spiritual awakening. The Yoga Sutras consist of 196 sutras (aphorisms) divided into four chapters (padas), each unveiling the essential principles and practices that lead the practitioner towards the ultimate goal of yoga – the state of Samadhi, a profound meditative absorption and union with the divine. From the ethical foundation of the Yamas and Niyamas to the practical techniques of asana and pranayama, each sutra weaves together a tapestry of wisdom that resonates across centuries, offering a timeless roadmap for seekers on the yogic path.

Samadhi Pada: The first chapter of the Yoga Sutras, Samadhi Pada, sets the foundation for the entire text by introducing the fundamental principles of yoga and defining its essence. It opens with the iconic sutra, "Atha yoganushasanam," which translates to "Now, the teachings of yoga are presented." This sutra emphasizes the significance of being present and ready to embark on the journey of self-discovery and spiritual evolution.

Patanjali introduces the concept of Chitta Vritti Nirodha, which means the cessation of the fluctuations of the mind. According to Patanjali, yoga is the process of calming the restless mind and attaining a state of stillness and clarity. He explains that the state of Samadhi, the ultimate goal of yoga, is achieved when the mind is free from distractions and attains a deep meditative absorption.

To achieve this state, Patanjali introduces the Eight Limbs of Yoga (Ashtanga Yoga), a systematic path that guides practitioners towards self-realization. These limbs include Yamas (ethical principles), Niyamas (self-disciplines), Asana (physical postures), Pranayama (breath control), Pratyahara (withdrawal of the senses), Dharana (concentration), Dhyana (meditation), and Samadhi (union).

Patanjali elucidates the five types of mental fluctuations (Vrittis) that disturb the mind and lead to suffering. These fluctuations are valid knowledge (Pramana), misconception (Viparyaya), imagination (Vikalpa), sleep (Nidra), and memory (Smriti). By understanding and transcending these Vrittis, practitioners can attain mental clarity and inner peace.

Sadhana Pada: The second chapter, Sadhana Pada, delves into the practical aspects of yoga and the means to attain a steady practice (Sadhana) that leads to spiritual growth. Patanjali highlights the importance of tapas (austerity), svadhyaya (self-study), and Ishvara pranidhana (surrender to a higher power) as essential components of the yogic journey.

He introduces the concept of Kriya Yoga, which consists of three components: Tapas (discipline and self-effort), Svadhyaya (self-study and contemplation of sacred texts), and Ishvara pranidhana (surrender to the divine). Kriya Yoga serves as a transformative practice that purifies the mind and leads to self-realization. Patanjali explores the obstacles (antarayas) that hinder progress on the yogic path, such as physical and mental ailments, doubt, laziness, and lack of focus. He offers guidance on how to overcome these obstacles and maintain unwavering commitment to the practice. The chapter also expounds on the concept of Ashtanga Yoga, the Eight-Limbed Yoga, elaborating on the first five limbs (Yamas, Niyamas, Asana, Pranayama, Pratyahara) and how they contribute to the process of inner purification and self-realization.

Vibhuti Pada: Vibhuti Pada, the third chapter, delves into the mystical aspects of yoga and the siddhis (extraordinary powers) that may arise as a result of advanced practice. Patanjali warns practitioners not to be distracted or attached to these siddhis but rather to stay focused on the ultimate goal of Samadhi and self-realization. The chapter highlights the power of concentration (Dharana) and the importance of directing the mind towards a single-pointed focus. By cultivating unwavering concentration, practitioners attain control over the mind and its tendencies. Patanjali explains the concept of Samyama, which is the combined practice of Dharana (concentration), Dhyana (meditation), and Samadhi (absorption). Through Samyama, practitioners gain profound insight into the object of meditation, leading to spiritual realization and the awakening of inner wisdom.

The chapter also introduces the concept of kleshas, the afflictions or sources of suffering that cloud the mind and lead to bondage. The five kleshas are avidya (ignorance), asmita (egoism), raga (attachment), dvesha (aversion), and abhinivesha (fear of death). By understanding and transcending these kleshas, seekers can attain freedom and liberation.

Kaivalya Pada: The final chapter, Kaivalya Pada, expounds on the state of Kaivalya, the ultimate liberation and freedom that arises when the individual self (Purusha) is liberated from the influence of Prakriti (the material world). In this state, the individual realizes their true nature and transcends the cycle of birth and death.

Patanjali describes the stages of spiritual realization and the journey towards Kaivalya. He emphasizes the importance of non-attachment and self-awareness in the process of self-realization.

The chapter also explores the concept of viveka (discrimination) and the importance of discerning between the eternal self (Purusha) and the impermanent material world (Prakriti). Through viveka, seekers can attain liberation from the cycles of suffering and rebirth.

Patanjali concludes the Yoga Sutras by emphasizing the significance of sustained practice and unwavering dedication to the path of yoga. He reminds practitioners that the journey of self-realization requires patience, perseverance, and deep inner longing for spiritual awakening.

In conclusion, the Yoga Sutras of Patanjali stand as a profound and timeless text that illuminates the path of yoga and unveils the essence of self-realization. From the foundational principles of ethical living to the practical techniques of meditation and concentration, each sutra weaves together a tapestry of wisdom that resonates across centuries, offering a timeless roadmap for seekers on the yogic path. As practitioners delve into the teachings of the Yoga Sutras, they are guided towards the ultimate goal of Samadhi, a state of profound meditative absorption and union with the divine. In the sanctuary of these ancient aphorisms, seekers discover the keys to unlock the treasures of inner peace, self-awareness, and spiritual liberation, enriching their lives with the profound wisdom that has guided humanity on its quest for self-realization for millennia.

What is the meaning of Asanas?

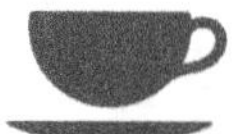

ASANAS, COMMONLY KNOWN as yoga postures, form an integral part of the ancient and profound practice of yoga. The term "asana" is derived from the Sanskrit root "as," which means "to sit" or "to be seated." However, the broader meaning of asanas transcends mere physical postures; it embodies a profound philosophy that weaves together the physical, mental, and spiritual aspects of the practitioner. Asanas are not merely exercises or stretches; they are sacred tools for self-discovery, mindfulness, and inner transformation.

At the physical level, asanas encompass a wide range of postures that nurture strength, flexibility, and balance in the body. From the grounding stability of Tadasana (Mountain Pose) to the graceful flow of Vinyasa sequences, each asana has its unique benefits for the body. Practicing asanas helps improve blood circulation, enhance joint mobility, and support the proper functioning of bodily systems. As the body moves through the postures, it releases tension, improves posture, and increases vitality.

Beyond the physical realm, asanas serve as portals to the mind, facilitating a deep state of mindfulness and presence. As practitioners flow through the sequences, they are encouraged to maintain a conscious awareness of their breath, sensations, and thoughts. This mindful presence cultivates a sense of grounded-ness, calms the mind, and enables the practitioner to be fully present in the moment.

At a subtler level, asanas are pathways to spiritual growth and self-realization. According to the ancient yogic philosophy, the human body is a temple for the soul (Atman). By practicing asanas with devotion and mindfulness, practitioners align their physical body with their higher self, fostering a deep sense of unity and interconnectedness.

Asanas are not about achieving perfect physical alignment; they are about exploring and understanding the body's limitations and possibilities. The journey of practicing asanas involves self-acceptance, self-compassion, and letting go of the ego's need for perfection. It is a journey of self-discovery and self-awareness, guiding practitioners to connect with their inner essence and embrace their authentic selves.

In the practice of asanas, the breath becomes the bridge between the physical and the spiritual realms. The synchronization of breath with movement (Vinyasa) infuses the practice with a meditative quality, calming the mind and allowing the practitioner to experience a sense of flow and harmony. As the breath becomes steady and controlled, the mind follows suit, transcending the constant chatter of thoughts and finding solace in the present moment.

Each asana carries its symbolism and unique energetic qualities. For instance, the heart-opening postures like Bhujangasana (Cobra Pose) and Ustrasana (Camel Pose) are associated with qualities of love, compassion, and vulnerability. Inversions, such as Sirsasana (Headstand) and Adho Mukha Vrksasana (Handstand), symbolize a shift in perspective and the ability to see things from a new angle. As practitioners embody these postures, they tap into the underlying energies and qualities they represent, transforming their practice into a meditative and transformative experience.

Asanas are also an expression of devotion and reverence towards the divine. Many asanas are named after animals, plants, sages, and celestial beings, symbolizing the connection between the physical and the spiritual realms. By embodying these asanas, practitioners honor the wisdom of nature and the divine within themselves.

In traditional Hatha Yoga, asanas were practiced to prepare the body for meditation. The physical postures helped release tension and restlessness, allowing the practitioner to sit comfortably for extended periods of meditation. Even today, the practice of asanas remains an essential foundation for meditation and inner exploration.

Asanas are not limited to a specific age, body type, or physical condition. They are accessible to everyone, regardless of their age or physical abilities. Yoga's inclusive nature embraces diversity and encourages practitioners to honour their bodies' unique needs and capacities. Modifications and variations are offered to accommodate different levels of experience and physical limitations, making yoga a practice that can be adapted to suit individual needs.

In the modern world, the practice of asanas has evolved and diversified, encompassing various yoga styles and traditions. From the dynamic and challenging sequences of Ashtanga Vinyasa Yoga to the gentle and therapeutic approach of Yin Yoga, each style offers a unique perspective on asana practice. Despite the diversity, the underlying essence of asanas remains constant - a journey of self-exploration, mindfulness, and spiritual growth.

The meaning of asanas extends far beyond physical postures; it embodies a holistic philosophy that weaves together the physical, mental, and spiritual dimensions of the practitioner. Asanas are sacred tools for self-discovery, mindfulness, and inner transformation, nurturing strength and flexibility in the body while calming the mind and fostering a deep sense of unity with the higher self. The practice of asanas is a journey of self-acceptance, self-awareness, and devotion, bridging the physical and spiritual realms through the breath and conscious presence. In the sanctuary of asanas, practitioners find solace, inspiration, and a profound connection with their inner essence, unlocking the treasures of self-realization and radiant well-being.

How to practice the yoga asanas (postures)

THE PROCESS OF DOING normal exercises which we did in school and doing asanas is the same. You have to warm up the body like you do in a gym, and not overstretch your body by doing excessive asanas, because the human body is the same and has the same hands, legs and other body parts whether you do yoga or do routing school PT exercises or gym. The effects on the body are going to be the same as all are different types of exercises not something magical or supernatural.

When you stop exercising or gym activity, pain starts building up in the body and the same applies to yoga. These need to be done regularly as the body gets programmed and if you stop them in between the body routine chances and the mind reacts with muscle pain and other effects.

Practicing yoga asanas (postures) is a transformative and enriching experience that nurtures the body, calms the mind, and uplifts the spirit. Whether you are a beginner or an experienced practitioner, the practice of asanas requires mindfulness, self-awareness, and a sense of devotion towards the process of self-discovery. Below are guidelines to help you cultivate a safe, effective, and meaningful asana practice:

Start with a Warm-Up: Before diving into the more intense postures, begin your practice with a gentle warm-up to prepare the body. Incorporate gentle stretches, joint rotations, and breath awareness to awaken the muscles and increase blood circulation.

Listen to Your Body: Yoga is not a competition; it is a journey of self-exploration. Pay attention to your body's needs and limitations. Respect your boundaries, and avoid pushing yourself into positions that cause pain or discomfort. Remember that everybody is unique, and your practice is a personal expression of self-care and self-compassion.

Breathe Mindfully: The breath is the cornerstone of the yoga practice. As you move through each posture, synchronize your breath with the movement. Practice Ujjayi breath (victorious breath) or natural deep breathing to create a sense of flow and calmness.

Focus on Alignment: Proper alignment is crucial for a safe and effective practice. Listen to the cues of your yoga teacher or use a mirror to check your alignment. Aligning your body correctly not only prevents injuries but also enhances the benefits of each pose.

Engage Core Muscles: In many postures, engaging the core muscles provides stability and support to the spine and enhances overall body awareness. Keep the abdominal muscles lightly engaged during your practice to protect the lower back and maintain balance.

Find Balance: Include a mix of standing, seated, twisting, back bending, forward bending, and balancing poses in your practice. Balancing the practice helps you strengthen and stretch different muscle groups, promoting overall harmony in the body.

Hold Poses Mindfully: Spend enough time in each posture to experience its effects fully. Avoid rushing through the practice; instead, savour each moment and find a balance between effort and ease.

Use Props Wisely: Yoga props such as blocks, straps, bolsters, and blankets can be valuable tools to support your practice. Props help in achieving proper alignment, especially for beginners or those with physical limitations.

Progress Gradually: If you are new to yoga or trying a challenging pose, progress step-by-step. Work with preparatory poses and gradually build strength and flexibility to move towards the more advanced postures.

Modify As Needed: Do not be afraid to modify poses to suit your body's needs. For instance, use a block under your hand in Trikonasana (Triangle Pose) if you cannot reach the floor. Modifying poses makes them accessible and safe for every practitioner.

Maintain a Regular Practice: Consistency is key to progress in yoga. Aim for a regular practice, even if it is a shorter session. A few minutes of daily practice can be more beneficial than sporadic, long sessions.

Honor Your Breath: If your breath becomes strained or irregular, it is an indication that you might be pushing yourself too hard. Come out of the pose or modify it to regain steady breathing.

Cultivate Mindfulness: Yoga is a moving meditation. Cultivate mindfulness by staying fully present during your practice. Observe your thoughts, sensations, and emotions without judgment, allowing yourself to be fully immersed in the present moment.

Embrace Rest and Savasana: After an intense practice, take time for relaxation and integration. Spend a few minutes in Savasana (Corpse Pose) to allow the body and mind to assimilate the benefits of the practice.

Seek Guidance: If you are new to yoga or exploring more advanced postures, seek guidance from a qualified yoga teacher. A skilled teacher can provide personalized adjustments, tips, and modifications to enhance your practice safely.

The practice of yoga asanas is a journey of self-discovery, self-awareness, and self-care. Embrace the essence of yoga by approaching your practice with mindfulness, patience, and compassion towards yourself. Listen to your body, honour its needs, and cultivate a sense of devotion towards your practice. As you flow through the postures with conscious breath and focused intention, you will experience the transformative power of yoga unfolding within you, enriching your life with a profound sense of well-being, balance, and inner harmony.

The different types of asanas and their benefits

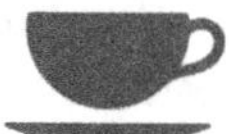

SOME OF THE ASANAS are similar to the PT exercises we are taught in schools. They include standing on one leg, stretching both legs and trying to touch them with our hands, bending backwards, forward, rotating left or right, moving head left or right alternatively, raising hangs up and down. These are the PT exercises we did at school.

In addition to these the asanas have sitting in a posture with both legs raised over each other and performing the up and down methods of PT exercises by keeping the legs intertwined while sitting in that posture. This is yoga and in this extra power is required and it stretches the muscles more than what happens in PT exercises. The asanas also include various breathing techniques while staying in the sitting posture with one leg kept over the other creating a unique experience of observing our breath consciously. The effect is similar to what we felt after running a long cross-country race, but getting the effect with lesser effort by the yoga sitting posture and deep breathing. It saves your time to run a long race to get the same effect and is less tiring. Writing a book itself is a PT exercise, Gym or asanas.

Below are different types of asanas along with their benefits:

Standing Asanas: Standing asanas form the foundation of a yoga practice, providing a stable base and fostering a sense of groundedness. They strengthen the legs, improve posture, and build overall body awareness. Examples include Tadasana (Mountain Pose), Virabhadrasana (Warrior Pose), and Trikonasana (Triangle Pose).

Forward Bending Asanas: Forward bending asanas promote introspection and relaxation, calming the mind and relieving stress. These poses stretch the hamstrings and lower back, and they massage the abdominal organs, aiding in digestion. Examples include Uttanasana (Standing Forward Bend) and Paschimottanasana (Seated Forward Bend).

Backbending Asanas: Backbends open the chest and heart center, enhancing the flow of energy and promoting emotional release. They improve spine flexibility and counteract the effects of prolonged sitting and slouching. Examples include Bhujangasana (Cobra Pose) and Ustrasana (Camel Pose).

Twisting Asanas: Twists detoxify the body, massaging the internal organs and improving digestion. These asanas also stimulate the spine's mobility and release tension in the back muscles. Examples include Ardha Matsyendrasana (Half Lord of the Fishes Pose) and Parivrtta Trikonasana (Revolved Triangle Pose).

Balancing Asanas: Balancing asanas cultivate focus, concentration, and a strong sense of presence. They build stability in the body and mind, enhancing overall coordination and proprioception. Examples include Vrikshasana (Tree Pose) and Bakasana (Crow Pose).

Inversion Asanas: Inversion asanas reverse the body's typical orientation, with the head below the heart. They promote blood circulation, stimulate the nervous system, and cultivate courage and mental clarity. Examples include Sirsasana (Headstand) and Sarvangasana (Shoulder Stand).

Core Strengthening Asanas: Core strengthening asanas target the muscles of the abdomen, lower back, and pelvis, providing stability and support to the spine. A strong core is essential for maintaining proper posture and preventing back pain. Examples include Navasana (Boat Pose) and Chaturanga Dandasana (Four-Limbed Staff Pose).

Hip Opening Asanas: Hip opening asanas release tension in the hips and lower back, where emotional and physical stress often accumulates. They also improve flexibility in the hip joints. Examples include Baddha Konasana (Butterfly Pose) and Eka Pada Rajakapotasana (Pigeon Pose).

Arm Balancing Asanas: Arm balances require strength, stability, and focus. They challenge practitioners to overcome fear and build confidence in their physical abilities. Arm balances also strengthen the upper body and core muscles. Examples include Bakasana (Crow Pose) and Pincha Mayurasana (Feathered Peacock Pose).

Restorative Asanas: Restorative asanas induce deep relaxation and reduce stress levels. They provide an opportunity for the body and mind to rejuvenate and restore balance. Examples include Balasana (Child's Pose) and Savasana (Corpse Pose).

Prone Asanas: Prone asanas are practiced lying face down, stretching the front of the body and strengthening the back muscles. They also improve posture and alleviate tension in the neck and shoulders. Examples include Bhujangasana (Cobra Pose) and Dhanurasana (Bow Pose).

Supine Asanas: Supine asanas are practiced lying on the back, allowing the body to relax and release tension. They promote a sense of surrender and peace. Examples include Supta Baddha Konasana (Reclining Bound Angle Pose) and Setu Bandhasana (Bridge Pose).

Benefits of Asanas

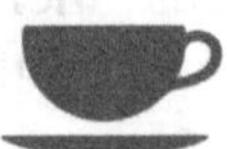

ASANAS IMPROVE STRENGTH, flexibility, and balance, enhancing overall physical fitness. They also improve posture, prevent injuries, and promote joint mobility. Regular practice of asanas supports weight management and contributes to cardiovascular health.

Asanas cultivate mindfulness, focus, and concentration, calming the mind and reducing stress and anxiety. They provide a sense of achievement and boost self-confidence. The meditative quality of asanas enhances self-awareness and emotional well-being.

Asanas are a means of preparing the body and mind for meditation, facilitating a deeper spiritual connection. They encourage the flow of prana (life force) through the body, promoting spiritual growth and self-realization.

Asanas stimulate the energy channels (nadis) and energy centers (chakras) in the body, promoting balanced energy flow. They awaken dormant energy and awaken the Kundalini, the spiritual energy located at the base of the spine.

Twists and inversions aid in detoxifying the body, stimulating the organs and promoting better elimination of waste and toxins. This cleansing effect revitalizes the body's systems and improves overall health.

The calming and relaxing effect of restorative asanas can improve the quality of sleep, helping practitioners experience more restful and rejuvenating nights.

Backbends and heart-opening asanas may lead to emotional release, helping practitioners process and release stored emotions.

The synchronization of breath with movement in asanas improves lung capacity and respiratory function, enhancing overall well-being.

Asanas foster a deep connection between the body and mind, promoting harmony and balance between physical, mental, and emotional aspects of the practitioner.

Regular practice of asanas increases flexibility and range of motion, reducing the risk of injuries.

Deep Breathing Technique: Pranayama

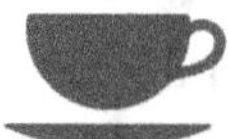

PRANAYAMA, THE ANCIENT yogic practice of deep breathing techniques, is a profound and transformative discipline that harnesses the power of the breath to calm the mind, revitalize the body, and connect with the essence of life force. The term "Pranayama" is derived from the Sanskrit words "Prana," meaning vital energy or life force, and "Ayama," meaning extension or expansion. Through conscious control and manipulation of the breath, Pranayama empowers practitioners to tap into the subtle energy within and unlock a vast array of physical, mental, and spiritual benefits. This ancient art of breathwork has been a cornerstone of yoga and meditation practices for millennia, offering seekers a gateway to inner peace, clarity, and spiritual awakening.

To begin the practice of Pranayama, find a comfortable seated position, with the spine erect and shoulders relaxed. Rest your hands on your knees or in a comfortable mudra (hand gesture). Gently close your eyes and bring your awareness to your breath. Observe the natural flow of your breath without trying to change it, noticing the sensations as the breath moves in and out of your body.

Diaphragmatic Breathing (Deergha Swasam or Three-Part Breath): Begin by taking a few deep breaths, filling your belly, ribcage, and chest with each inhalation. As you exhale, release the breath from the chest, ribcage, and belly. Continue this deep three-part breath, focusing on extending the breath and creating a sense of fullness and expansion with each inhale and complete release with each exhale. This technique calms the nervous system, increases lung capacity, and reduces stress and anxiety.

Nadi Shodhana (Alternate Nostril Breathing): Bring your right thumb to the right nostril and close it gently. Inhale deeply and slowly through the left nostril. At the end of the inhale, close the left nostril with your right ring finger and release the right nostril. Exhale slowly and completely through the right nostril. Inhale deeply through the right nostril, close it with the right thumb, and release the left nostril. Exhale through the left nostril. This completes one round. Continue for several rounds, focusing on the smooth and even flow of breath through both nostrils. Nadi Shodhana balances the flow of energy in the body and calms the mind, promoting mental clarity and harmony.

Ujjayi Breathing (Victorious Breath): Inhale deeply through the nose, slightly constricting the back of the throat to create a soft, ocean-like sound. Exhale through the nose with the same gentle constriction. Continue the Ujjayi breath throughout your practice, using it to anchor your awareness and deepen your connection to the present moment. Ujjayi breathing builds heat in the body, enhances concentration, and increases mindfulness.

Kapalabhati (Skull Shining Breath): Sit comfortably with a straight spine and take a deep inhale. As you exhale, forcefully and quickly contract your abdominal muscles to push the breath out in short bursts. The inhalation happens naturally as the belly relaxes. Start with a few rounds and gradually increase the pace. After completing the rounds, take a few deep breaths to normalize your breathing. Kapalabhati detoxifies the body, invigorates the nervous system, and enhances mental clarity.

Bhramari Pranayama (Bee Breath): Close your eyes and gently close your ears with your thumbs, your eyes with your index fingers, and your nostrils with your middle fingers. Inhale deeply, and as you exhale, create a soft humming sound like a bee. Feel the vibrations of the sound soothing your mind and calming your nervous system. Repeat for several rounds. Bhramari Pranayama relieves stress, anxiety, and tension, promoting a sense of inner peace and tranquillity.

Sheetali Pranayama (Cooling Breath): Roll your tongue into a tube shape or purse your lips, creating a small "O" shape. Inhale deeply through the rolled tongue or pursed lips, drawing in cool air. Close your mouth and exhale through the nose. Continue for several rounds, enjoying the cooling sensation of the breath. Sheetali Pranayama reduces body heat, calms the mind, and alleviates stress.

Sheetkari Pranayama (Hissing Breath): Gently clench your teeth together, keeping your lips apart. Inhale slowly and deeply through your teeth, making a hissing sound. Close your mouth and exhale through the nose. Repeat for several rounds. Sheetkari Pranayama has a cooling effect on the body, reduces anger, and soothes the nervous system.

Sama Vritti (Equal Breathing): Inhale to a count of four, hold the breath for a count of four, exhale to a count of four, and hold the breath out for a count of four. This creates a balanced and even breath pattern, promoting mental clarity and focus.

Bhastrika Pranayama (Bellows Breath): Sit comfortably with your back straight and shoulders relaxed. Take a deep inhalation and exhale forcefully through the nose, followed by rapid and powerful inhalations and exhalations. The breath is driven by the movement of the diaphragm, with the chest remaining relatively still. After completing several rounds, take a few deep breaths to return to normal breathing. Bhastrika Pranayama increases oxygen intake, invigorates the body, and builds respiratory strength.

Brahmari Pranayama (Humming Bee Breath): Sit comfortably and place your hands on your face with your fingers on your closed eyelids, thumbs covering your ears, and the rest of your fingers resting on your cheeks. Inhale deeply, and as you exhale, create a soft humming sound like a bee. Feel the vibrations of the sound soothing your mind and calming your nervous system. Repeat for several rounds. Brahmari Pranayama relieves stress, anxiety, and tension, promoting a sense of inner peace and tranquillity.

Agni Prasana (Breath of Fire): Sit comfortably with your spine straight and hands on your knees. Inhale deeply through your nose, and as you exhale, forcefully contract your abdominal muscles to push the breath out in short bursts. The inhalation happens naturally as the belly relaxes. Continue this rhythmic and rapid breath for a few rounds, followed by deep breathing to normalize your breath. Agni Prasana generates heat in the body, increases metabolism, and activates the solar plexus.

Incorporate Pranayama into your daily yoga practice or as a standalone practice to experience its profound benefits. Regular and consistent Pranayama practice can lead to a profound transformation, promoting physical well-being, emotional balance, and spiritual awakening. Remember that Pranayama is not merely a mechanical exercise but a sacred art of conscious breathing

Basically meditation, yoga, PT exercises, Gym, swimming and other methods remove tension, stress, anxiety, become positive, make us feel energised, reduce illness and diseases and offer a host of other benefits.

Holidays and Pilgrimage

WHEN WE TRAVEL ON HOLIDAYS, it allows us to escape from the stressful life of cities. While it is difficult to leave our jobs in cities, the holidays help us to escape the cities for a short time.

These holidays and pilgrimage are another form of meditation and yoga. At the time of holidays, you are conscious of what you eat and where you eat. You are conscious on the cost of hotels and save on the stay and meals as much as possible. This is because you get more time for yourself, and save time which you had earlier given for work related activities which take up 80 % of your mind. Going away a longer distance from you work place also gives you relief from the thoughts which acted on you related to your everyday activities and more than half of the unwanted thoughts go away.

The reason we give machines and computer a rest during the night is that they cool down and even machines accumulate stress as it is a mechanical property. Stress is mechanical, the more we work the more stress stores inside machines or our bodies.

Beyond the conventional perception of these experiences of holidays as mere leisure pursuits or religious endeavours, they beckon us to embark on a sacred journey of inner exploration and self-discovery. Each holiday, whether amidst serene beaches or majestic mountains, and every pilgrimage to sacred sites, becomes a canvas for weaving the threads of mindfulness, meditation, and yoga into the fabric of our lives.

When we embark on a holiday with a mindful lens, we venture into the heart of awareness, allowing us to witness life with fresh eyes and an open heart. From the moment we set foot in a new environment, we become attuned to the beauty of the surroundings the sights, the sounds, the scents. Every breath becomes a gateway to the present, as we immerse ourselves in the symphony of existence.

The sun-kissed beaches, the serene forests, or the tranquil meadows each destination offers unique opportunities for meditation and yoga. As we gaze at the vastness of the ocean or the grandeur of the mountains, we are reminded of the infinite nature of consciousness. We become aware of our place in the tapestry of existence, connecting with the vastness of the universe within ourselves.

In the midst of holidays, we find ourselves liberated from the shackles of our regular routine. Amidst the luxury of time and space, we have the privilege of immersing ourselves in the art of stillness. As the sun rises and sets, and the moon casts its luminous glow, we find solace in silence and stillness, becoming one with the rhythm of nature.

With each passing moment, we allow our minds to settle, like ripples on a tranquil lake. We embrace the ebb and flow of thoughts without judgment, simply observing them as they come and go. This is the essence of meditation – witnessing the ceaseless dance of the mind and finding the anchor of stillness within.

Holidays provide an opportunity to explore quietness beyond sitting in quietude. From savouring a delightful meal to taking a leisurely stroll along the shore, every moment becomes an invitation to practice mindfulness. Mindful eating automatically happens, we need not do meditation or yoga to learn mindful eating.

Yoga, too, finds its expression in every movement, every breath. The asanas become a symphony of grace, fluidity, and strength, as we embrace the dance of body and breath. Whether it's a morning flow on the beach or a gentle stretch under the stars, yoga becomes an embodied meditation, aligning mind, body, and spirit.

On holidays, our senses come alive as we bask in the abundance of sensory experiences. The touch of the sand beneath our feet, the taste of exotic cuisines, the fragrance of wildflowers in the air – each sensation becomes an opportunity to cultivate mindfulness. We savour every moment, fully immersed in the present, as if tasting the nectar of life itself. This itself is meditation and it is in humans for 10,000 years and meditation did not discover it. It was discovered by Nature.

The Healing Power of Nature: Nature is our greatest ally in the pursuit of happiness and peace. The serene landscapes, the awe-inspiring vistas, and the vibrant flora and fauna awaken a sense of wonder within us. We become attuned to the beauty and interconnectedness of all living beings, recognizing our role as custodians of this precious planet.

The Alchemy of Relaxation: Holidays are an opportune time to indulge in relaxation and self-care. From indulging in spa treatments to soaking in a warm bath, we surrender to the alchemy of relaxation. We honour our bodies as temples of the soul, embracing rest and rejuvenation as essential components of our holistic well-being.

The Dance of Inner Exploration: In the canvas of holidays, we embark on a journey of inner exploration, unearthing the treasures that lie within. We come face to face with our fears and limitations, gently releasing them with compassion. We cultivate self-compassion, embracing ourselves as imperfect yet infinitely worthy beings. We don't need meditation or yoga to tell us these things. They are only daily exercises as it is not possible for us to go on holidays frequently.

Connecting with the Sacred: As we traverse the landscapes of holidays, we encounter sacred spaces that evoke a sense of reverence within us. Temples, monasteries, or natural wonders each place carries a unique energy, inviting us to connect with the sacredness of life. These spaces, become a spiritual pilgrimage, drawing us closer to the divine essence that permeates all of creation. Nature is God and, God is creation.

The Power of Intention: Holidays empower us to set powerful intentions for our lives. As we take a step back from the cacophony of our routines, we gain clarity on what truly matters to us. We find the courage to align our actions with our deepest values, paving the way for a more purposeful and fulfilling life.

Cultivating Gratitude: Gratitude becomes our constant companion on holidays. We acknowledge the abundance in our lives, embracing the blessings that surround us. From the warmth of the sun to the laughter of loved ones, we bathe in the river of gratitude, discovering that every moment is an opportunity for thankfulness. By going on holidays, we treat ourselves for doing lot of hard work and reward ourselves. By doing meditation and yoga, we are trying to achieve the same thing but there is no reward such as holidays and pilgrimage which is needed to reward yourself and feel good.

Bringing Mindful Holidays into Everyday Life: As we bid farewell to holidays, we carry the essence of mindfulness, meditation, and yoga back into our daily lives. We recognize that holidays are not isolated events but a state of being – a way of living fully and authentically. We infuse our routines with moments of stillness, mindful movement, and self-compassion.

Mindful Eating: During the holidays we experience mindful eating. One of the most profound ways to integrate mindfulness into everyday life is through mindful eating it is basic thing and we don't need meditation or yoga to tell us this. We experience mindful eating in our holidays when we try to save on costs of eating and choose the food we eat in those places. We savour each bite, fully present in the sensory experience of eating. We appreciate the nourishment that food provides, cultivating a deeper connection with the sustenance that fuels our bodies in our holidays.

Mindful Movement: Beyond the meditation or yoga, we must infuse mindfulness into our daily movement. Whether it's walking, jogging, or even commuting, we become present in every step we take. The simple act of breathing becomes a reminder to return to the present moment, anchoring us in the here and now. Breathing is a natural thing and we are only air inside the body.

Mindful Relationships: Mindful holidays teach us the art of connection – not just with ourselves but with others. We carry this wisdom into our relationships, listening with full attention, and embracing the essence of compassion. We cultivate empathy and understanding, nurturing our connections with authenticity and vulnerability.

A Journey of Lifelong Growth: As we weave the tapestry of mindful holidays into our lives, we recognize that this is not a destination but an eternal journey. Meditation and yoga become our steadfast companions, guiding us through the ebbs and flows of life. Each moment becomes an opportunity for inner growth and self-discovery.

In the sanctuary of holidays, we realize that we are not separate from the vast tapestry of existence. We are interconnected with all living beings and the rhythms of the universe. Our journey becomes a celebration of oneness – an ode to the infinite nature of consciousness.

In the holidays, we become the co-creators of our destiny, dancing to the rhythm of our own heartbeats. Every step we take becomes a pilgrimage, every breath a meditation. Holidays become an opportunity to return to the essence of our being, to rediscover the sacredness of life, and to embrace the dance of existence with grace and gratitude.

As we journey through the landscape of mindful holidays, we unveil the secret that these experiences are not confined to a specific time or space. They are woven into the very fabric of our souls, guiding us on the path of self-discovery and spiritual awakening. The sacredness of life reveals itself in every moment, every breath, and every heartbeat.

Holidays are an eternal reminder of the beauty and depth that lies within each experience. May it inspire us to embrace every holiday as a sacred pilgrimage, a chance to connect with our true essence and the interconnectedness of all existence. And may we carry the wisdom of mindfulness, meditation, and yoga into the tapestry of our lives, weaving a symphony of presence and purpose in every breath we take.

Meditation, Yoga and Exercises are good for life, but we also need relaxation and contact with nature.

Exchanging Holidays with relatives

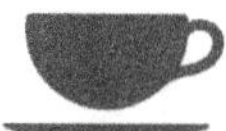

THE MIND AS SUCH CANNOT be controlled and meditation is temporary, unless you do it for a long time till your mind gets programmed to control thoughts which are coming from everywhere. Holidays allow you to escape from unwanted thoughts but are short lived and you gain new thoughts on coming back. You will need holidays every year provide you can afford them or exchange places by going to relatives and calling them to your place. This can save on costs.

This is a new method which I am suggesting although it is partially followed by some of us. We can either share the costs or pay the relatives for staying at their places. This method will become common in future as hotels and eating on holidays becomes costly, people will not be able to afford long holidays. In the old times, we did practise them when there were less hotels, we sent family members to places of relatives to stay which is much safer and the relatives also act as guides, helping with locations one can visit.

These give you the same effects which you want from meditation, yoga, other mind and body calming methods.

Fasting

FASTING IS ALSO IMPORTANT, as during fasting lot of unwanted chemicals get released form our body. Fasting is particularly good for overweight people, but they lose the benefits of fasting because they eat more after doing it. Poor people do mindful eating as they have limited food and need to survive on very little they have and they savour each and every bite. Thet is why you see them having good bodies and figure. Only problem is they suffer from malnutrition as they are not able to buy all kinds of foods.

But we eat all kinds of foods leading to our body filled with unwanted chemicals and excess nutrients and this also puts a load on our thighs and joints and the body needs to work more to digest all of it. If you are unable to exercise, do meditation or yoga, you can simply practise fasting. It helps to improve your digestion system and may even cure some illnesses.

Body pain, stiffness, diseases are related to unwanted contents in your body and it may be micro-organisms or chemicals or both of them. When you fast, these get purged out of your body and it may help to cure some of the diseases. Unwanted dead cells also get removed during fasting. That is why some people recommend fasting with meditation and yoga, because it is fasting which is giving more benefit than meditation and yoga. Yoga is only for consuming the excess energy within your body by stretching and exercising.

Taking a Bath

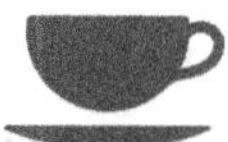

TAKING A BATH IS ANOTHER way of relaxation. It is not possible for everyone to take a bath daily as some people get sick while taking a bath and others feel uncomfortable or their bodies become cold. Therefore, they prefer to take a hot bath. That is why salt baths, spring baths, steam baths are popular but they are costly. We spend on these hot baths as we are lazy to do them in our own house are lack the facilities.

If we were to take bath regularly, it would reduce the time we spend in doing meditation, yoga, exercises or going to the gym. Everyone knows we need to take a bath after an exercise or going to the gym, but in meditation and yoga, preferably the bath is taken first. It is exactly opposite as meditation and yoga don't produce sweating as much as exercising or gym. In these methods the toxins go out of body due to sweating and then we bath to remove the toxins on our skins.

For meditation and yoga since there is little or no sweating, we need to fast, so the toxins get removed trough digestion or through the bowels. Without mediation and yoga also, the toxins can remove simply by fasting.

Too much hot water or steam bath can result in your boy paining a lot. A bath helps to remove the germs on your skin which are also responsible for pain, stress, uneven mind and unwanted thoughts. All this are a combination of several factors including pollution and also living in a stressful environment such as daily noises, disturbances in family and neighbourhoods and so on which are unavoidable. A bath helps you get relief from all this factors and you will not require meditation or yoga to cleanse yourself of environmental causes and factors.

The decision to take a bath before or after meditation and yoga ultimately depends on personal preference and individual needs. Both approaches have their benefits, and it's essential to find what works best for you and aligns with your practice. Here are some considerations for each option:

Before Meditation and Yoga: Taking a bath before meditation and yoga can help you relax and prepare your body and mind for practice. A warm bath can soothe muscles and release tension, making it easier to sit or move comfortably during your practice. The calming effect of a bath can also help to quiet the mind, making it easier to enter a meditative state.

Additionally, a bath before practice can be a ritual of self-care and purification. It can be an opportunity to cleanse yourself both physically and mentally, setting a clear intention for your meditation and yoga session.

After Meditation and Yoga: Taking a bath after meditation and yoga can be a way to continue the sense of relaxation and rejuvenation that comes from your practice. It can help you unwind further and provide a sense of reward for the efforts you put into your meditation and yoga session.

Moreover, a bath after practice can be a form of self-care and a way to take care of your body. It can help ease any soreness or stiffness that may have arisen during your yoga practice, allowing your muscles to recover and relax.

Ultimately, the decision on when to take a bath should be based on what feels most comfortable and beneficial for you. Some people may prefer to take a bath before their practice to set the tone for relaxation and focus, while others may find it more enjoyable and soothing to take a bath after their practice as a way to wind down and refresh.

As you integrate meditation and yoga into your daily routine, you'll discover what works best for you. Listen to your body and honour your needs, allowing your practice to be a reflection of self-care and mindfulness in every aspect of your life.

Don't miss out!

Click the button below and you can sign up to receive emails whenever Jagdish Krishanlal Arora publishes a new book. There's no charge and no obligation.

Also by Jagdish Krishanlal Arora

WordPress Design and Development
World War III
Travellers Guide to Mount Kailash
Become a Better Writer With Creative Writing
Emerging Trends in Carbon Emission Reduction
India Independence Through Non Violence
Copyright, Patents, Trademarks and Trade Secret Laws
Decoding CHATGPT and Artificial Intelligence
The Untold Story of Diana and Prince Charles
Time Travel
How to Lose Weight Quickly
Subconcious Programming
Productive Healthcare Management
Arandor
The Attic's Secrets
Risks Associated with Artifical Intelligence and Robotics
Children of the Magic Realm
The Code of Hammurabi
Large Language Models - LLMs
Cyber Security
Romantic Noveels Collection
Data Science – Neural Networks, Deep Learning, LLMs and Power BI
Manusmriti
Planet Earth
Space, Time and Matter
Ukraine vs Russia
King's Love
Married to A Disabled Billionaire CEO
THE Ukraine Ceasefire Agreement and History
The New York Archives
World War IV: Russia Vs United States
God was Created by Early Human Civilizations

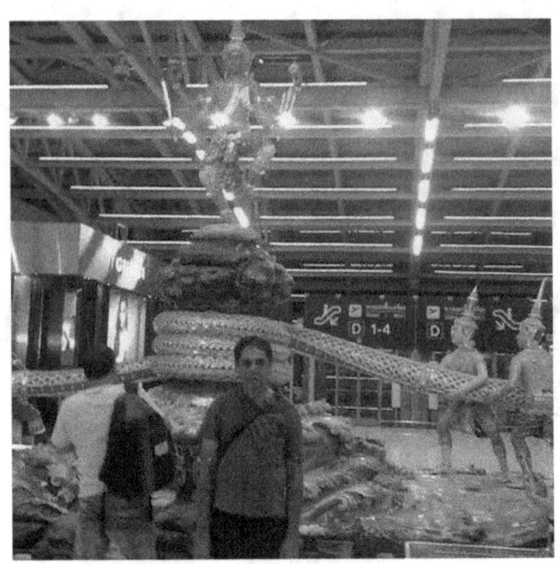

About the Author

As an author, with over 60+ books, Jagdish Krishanlal Arora continues to contribute to literature and education, touching the lives of readers across the globe. His books are widely appreciated for their clarity, insight, and ability to cater to a variety of interests. While he maintains a relatively low public profile, his extensive catalog of works speaks volumes about his dedication to knowledge-sharing and intellectual exploration.